INTERMITTENT FASTING FOR WOMEN OVER 50

The Complete Beginners Guide for Aging Women to Reset Metabolism | Learn The Best Lifestyle for Losing Weight, Eating Healthy, and Increase Your Energy

Grace Rogers

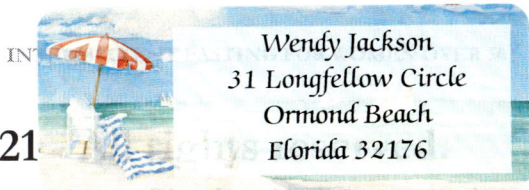

Table Of Contents

Introduction

Many people are living longer and have more opportunities to enjoy life. This is true for many women that are over 50 years of age. However, as they grow older, these women may experience changes in their body such as hormonal imbalances and metabolic syndrome.

Their bodies change which may cause them to experience health issues as they go through menopause. When women enter menopause, the body stops producing the same amount of estrogen in their 20s and 30s. Estrogen helps maintain bone density and can reduce problems during menopause, such as hot flashes and night sweats.

No matter what stage of life a woman is in, there are always changes that occur, causing imbalances in hormones and metabolism. Women who live a healthy lifestyle by eating a balanced diet and exercising regularly will experience fewer problems as they age.

However, most women over 50 have not embraced this ideal way of living or have ignored it completely because of family obligations or other things that occupy their time. It becomes more challenging for them to make time to exercise and eat the right foods. Many times, it leads to changes in their bodies, which leads to unnecessary health problems.

A healthy lifestyle and regular exercise can help prevent serious health problems. Still, it may not be enough to counter the effects of aging on hormones, weight, circulation, or energy levels. In addition to exercise and a healthy diet, Intermittent Fasting can help promote weight loss, blood pressure control, improve cognitive function, and reduce inflammation.

It is one of the effective ways to help improve health and well-being. It improves sleep quality, increases energy levels and mood. It's also a great way to boost metabolism and lose weight quickly in men and women. People who practice intermittent fasting often get the side effects of detoxification and cleansing.

Many women may have already experienced or are experiencing hormonal changes, stress, or depression. As women age, they are more susceptible to hormone imbalances, changing the body's metabolism and weight loss efforts. Women over 50 who fast can help improve their overall well-being and the health of their bodies. There are several benefits to fasting.

It improves overall health by removing toxins and excess water from the body. It also increases the ability to utilize micronutrients and nutrients. It improves muscle mass and reduces the amount of fat in the body.

Intermittent fasting is not just for weight loss but can also be used to treat many different diseases. It is beneficial in treating metabolic diseases, cancer, diabctcs, cardiovascular disease, neurological disorders, and many more.

This guide goes over the benefits of intermittent fasting, including how it can be helpful to lose weight, maintain a healthy weight and improve health. In addition, it provides information on when women should fast and ways to monitor how they feel during a fast. Suggestions for fasting include the different types of intermittent fasting and the health benefits it offers.

This also provides tips and advice on intermittent fasting that you can incorporate into your lifestyle. You will learn different ways to implement intermittent fasting into your routine and what it does to the body during a fast. You can easily follow this guide, and it doesn't require many changes in your lifestyle.

Chapter 1. A Guide to Intermittent Fasting

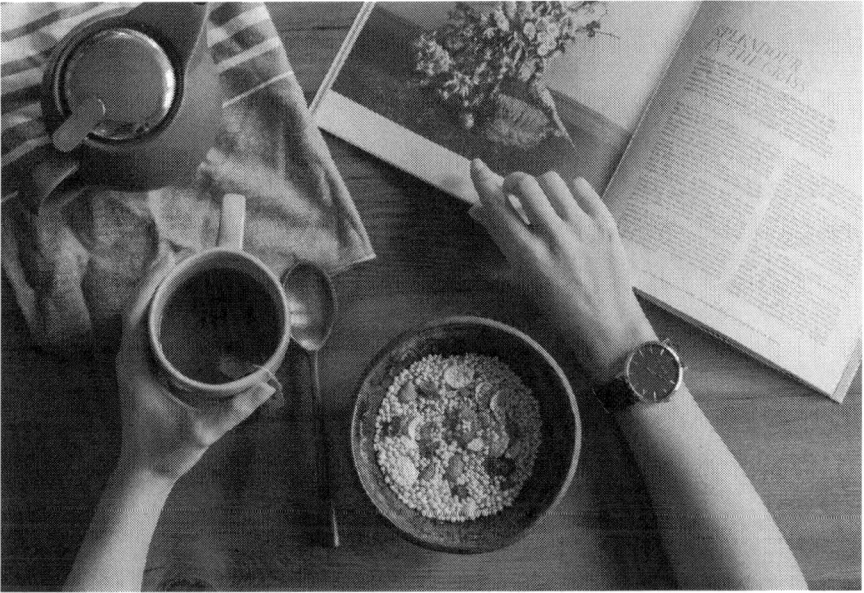

What Is Intermittent Fasting?

Intermittent fasting isn't an eating routine. It's a way of eating. It's a method for planning your meal so that you benefit from them. It doesn't change what you eat. It changes when you eat. This is an unconventional way to lose weight without having to eat crazy things or reduce calories to zero. Indeed, often you'll attempt to keep your calories at a similar level when you start discontinuous fasting. The vast majority eat greater suppers during a shorter period.

Additionally, it is a decent method to keep bulk on while getting lean. With all that stated, the major reason individuals attempt this kind of fasting is to lose fat. Intermittent fasting is perhaps the least complex procedure we have for dropping terrible weight while keeping the great load because it requires almost no conduct change. This is an excellent thing since it implies intermittent fasting falls into the class of basic enough that you'll do it, however, significant enough that it will have any effect.

How Does Intermittent Fasting Work?

Your body is in the fed state when it is processing and retaining nourishment.

Regularly, the fed state begins when you start eating and goes on for 3 to 5 hours as your body processes and retains the nourishment you just ate. It is more challenging for your body to consume fat because your insulin levels are high in the fed state. After that period, your body goes into what is known as the post-absorptive state, which is only an extravagant method for saying that your body isn't handling a feast. The post-absorptive state goes on until 8 to 12 hours after your last supper, which is the point at which you enter the fasted state.

It is much simpler for your body to consume fat in a fasted state because your insulin levels are low. At the point when you're in the fasted state, your body can consume fat that has been out of reach during the fed state. Since we don't enter the fasted state until 12 hours after our last supper, it's uncommon that our bodies are right now in this state.

This is why numerous individuals who start intermittent fasting will lose fat without changing what they eat, the amount they eat, or how regularly they work out. Fasting places your body in a fat-consuming state that you once were in a while, making it during a typical eating plan.

While it might be a mainstream pattern in the eating regimen world nowadays, those attempting to get thinner or improve their general wellbeing should realize that it tends to be a challenging arrangement to stick to. This is because the methodology shifts back and forth between times of fasting and non-fasting during a specific timeframe.

What Can I Eat While Intermittent Fasting?

You should stop consuming hard things on the system until the body knows that you aren't stressed and are just eating less often. Some individuals are certain that such foods irritate their stomachs more than others. If you have an issue with those ingredients, you can stop them when you first start eating again.

In general, we've discovered that these foods (and drinks) are the most difficult for people to eat while they're breaking their fast, while some people handle them fine:

- Nut butter and nuts
- Seed butter and seeds
- Vegetables cruciferous, raw
- Eggs
- Dairy products
- Alcohol
- Few may experience trouble digesting red meat or certain types of red meat on special occasions.

You should be able to eat the food mentioned here without trouble within six hours of breaking your fast.

- Make sure you're well-hydrated before you begin.
- Begin your meal with a cup of chopped parsley with tomatoes and cucumber salad. When desired, a tablespoon of extra virgin olive oil may be added.
- Keep your protein sources to poultry or fish to be healthy. They can be fried in fat, and the skin of the chicken can be eaten. Try to keep the protein consumption to no more than the scale and thickness of your palm.
- Complete the remainder of the plate with non-starchy, above-ground veggies fried in healthy fats such as avocado, cocoa butter, butter, or clarified butter.
- If you're ever hungry, add avocado at the end of your meal.

Intermittent Fasting Benefits

Intermittent fasting will help you lose weight while still lowering the chance of contracting a variety of diseases.

Heart Health

The main cause of death in the world is heart failure. High blood pressure, higher LDL cholesterol, and high triglyceride levels are three of the most common risks for cardiac failure.

Intermittent fasting reduced blood pressure by 6 percent in only eight weeks in a sample of sixteen obese men and women. According to the same report, intermittent fasting also reduced LDL cholesterol by 25percent or triglycerides by 32%. The evidence for a correlation between intermittent fasting and lower LDL cholesterol and triglycerides, on the other hand, is mixed.

Four weeks of intermittent fasting over the Islamic holiday of Ramadan did not result in a decrease in LDL cholesterol or triglycerides, according to a survey of 40 normal-weight individuals. Until researchers completely comprehend the impact of intermittent fasting on cardiac health, higher-quality experiments with more rigorous methods are needed.

Diabetes

Intermittent fasting will also help you treat your diabetes and lower your chances of contracting it. Intermittent fasting, including prolonged calorie restriction, tends to reduce some diabetes risk factors. It mostly accomplishes this by lowering insulin levels and decreasing insulin tolerance.

Six months of intermittent fasting cut insulin levels by 29% and insulin tolerance by 19% in a randomized controlled trial of more than 100 overweight or obese women. The amounts of blood sugar stayed unchanged.

Furthermore, intermittent fasting for 8–12 weeks has been found to decrease insulin levels by 20–31percent and blood glucose levels by 3–6percent in people with pre-diabetes, a disease wherein blood sugar levels are high but not severe enough to make a diagnosis.

In terms of blood sugar, though, intermittent fasting might not be as effective for females as males. A small study showed that women's blood sugar balance deteriorated throughout 22 days of alterative fasting, although men's blood sugar levels were unaffected. Considering this risk factor, the decrease in insulin and insulin tolerance will possibly reduce the incidence of diabetes, particularly in pre-diabetic individuals.

Weight Loss

When performed correctly, intermittent fasting can be an easy and efficient way to reduce weight since short-term fasts can let you eat fewer calories and lose weight. Several reports have found that intermittent fasting is just as successful as conventional calorie-restricted diets for weight loss in the short term.

Intermittent fasting resulted in an overall weight reduction of 15 lbs. (6.8 kg) over 3–12 months, according to a 2018 study of research in overweight adults. According to another study, for 3–24 weeks, intermittent fasting decreased body weight by 3–8% in overweight or obese individuals.

According to the report, participants' waist circumference decreased by 3–7% during the same period. It's worth noting that the long-term consequences of intermittent fasting on female weight loss are also unknown.

Intermittent starvation seems to help with weight reduction in the short term. Though, the amount you lose can most definitely be determined by how many calories you eat during non-fasting hours and how long you stick to the lifestyle.

It May Help You Eat Less

Transitioning to intermittent fasting may help you eat less naturally. According to one report, when young men's food consumption was limited to a four-hour duration, they consumed 650 fewer calories per day.

Another research looked at the impact of a lengthy, 36-hour fast on the eating patterns of 24 active men and women. Despite eating more calories on the post-fast day, participants' overall calorie balance fell by 1,900 calories, a substantial decrease.

Is Intermittent Fasting Safe?

Many women tend to be healthy by using modified forms of intermittent fasting. On the other hand, various studies have shown that fasting days will trigger hunger, mood fluctuations, loss of focus, decreased stamina, headaches, and bad breath. Women's menstrual cycles have also been said to have ceased while on an intermittent fasting diet, according to several reports on the internet.

Before attempting intermittent fasting, contact the doctor if you have a medical problem. Medical advice is especially relevant for women who:

- Also had an eating problem in the past.
- Suffer from low blood pressure daily or have diabetes.
- They are underweight, malnutrition, and deficient in nutrients.
- Are you expecting a child, are you breastfeeding, or are you planning to conceive?

Suffer from infertility or have a diagnosis of anemia (missed periods). There is a lot of evidence to back up the medicinal effects of fasting. Improved cellular fitness, improved metabolic indicators, and weight reduction are also possible health advantages.

Intermittent fasting causes weight loss in women, but it doesn't cause much further weight loss than a calorie deficiency overall, according to studies. On the other hand, the structure of IF allows it possible for certain people to limit their food consumption.

Intermittent fasting will also help you lose weight. Blood sugar (glucose) increases when we feed, and insulin is discharged to transport sugar to our body for energy. Excess glucose is quickly processed. If you go 10-16 hours without eating, your body can begin to use fat reserves for power.

Cellular repair happens in a fasted condition, according to research, and has been attributed to enhanced survival, lower cancer risk, lower inflammation, and better metabolism. However, several of the experiments are conducted on livestock, and further research on women is needed.

There's still new evidence that feeding in time with your circadian clock helps you avoid chronic diseases. In other terms, you are limiting overnight feeding to eating within a 6–10-hour window throughout the day when it's light outside.

Chapter 2. Menopause and Intermittent Fasting

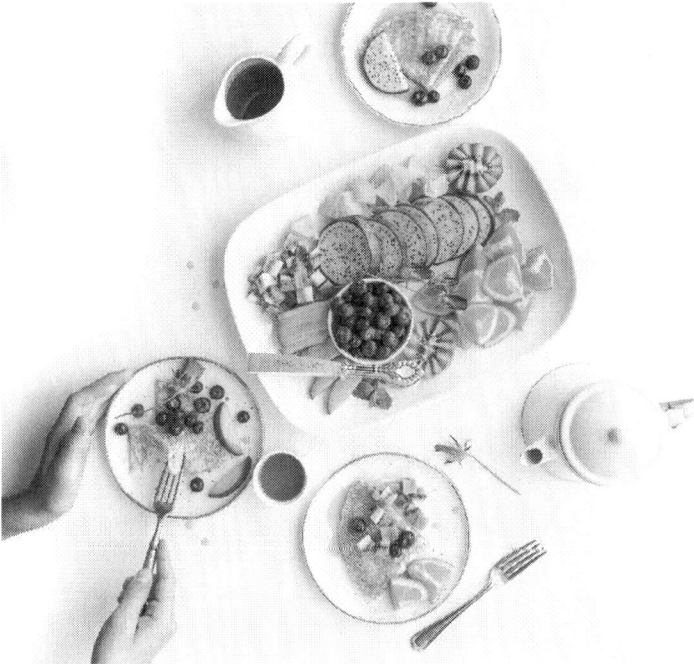

During the premenopausal and postmenopausal periods, a woman faces various health problems. These have a major impact on her quality of living. Numerous medical disciplines have used fasting as a remedy for a wide range of diseases since ancient times. However, even though research supports its clinical effectiveness, it is rarely used today as an intervention technique. Instead, it is limited in the popular imagination to a superstitious or religious regimen rather than a scientific practice.

Fasting plays an essential role in women's well-being throughout their lives. However, broader randomized control trials have been found to justify these benefits more extensively. The bulk of the trials available have significant drawbacks, like human studies and clinical trials conducted with small sample sizes.

In addition, fasting trials are hindered by ethical concerns over assigning humans to fast over long periods. Future research should focus on bridging this gap by developing medically controlled fasting methods that yield more data. Meanwhile, fasting can be recommended as a healthy and medically beneficial practice and a dietary regimen that can significantly improve women's health.

What is Menopause?

When a woman enters her 40s and 50s, her sex hormone levels begin to decrease spontaneously when the ovaries stop releasing estrogen and progesterone, which causes menstruation to stop.

Menopause is described as a woman not having a period for 12 consecutive months, but amenorrhea is far from the only symptom of the transition.

Hot flashes, vaginal dryness, nausea, reduced libido, brain fog, exhaustion, chill bumps, night sweats, mood swings, and an elevated risk of heart disease are some of the signs of menopause, which can vary from person to person. Certain women often experience a noticeable difference in metabolism, which usually slows when estrogen and progesterone levels become erratic, leading to weight gain.

Women may become less receptive to insulin after menopause. They may have difficulty consuming sugar and processed carbohydrates. This metabolic transition is known as insulin resistance and is frequently accompanied by exhaustion and sleeping problems.

Many women find menopause frightening; they can no longer recognize their bodies, while symptoms like unexpected weight gain and brain fog may cause anxiety, confusion, rage, stress, and depression.

Fortunately, women could use intermittent fasting as a method to help them navigate the confusing and worrying process of menopause. If you're experiencing nausea, excess weight, or insulin sensitivity due to menopause, you may want to try it.

Weight gain is aided by intermittent fasting. Fasting improves insulin sensitivity and allows the body to absorb sugar and carbohydrates more efficiently, lowering the risk of heart disease, diabetes, and some other metabolic disorders.

Fasting has been demonstrated to boost self-esteem, reduce depression, and stress, and promote positive psychological changes. In animal research, fasting has been found to help shield brain cells from trauma, remove waste products, and restore and improve bodily performance.

Symptoms of Menopause and Intermittent Fasting as a Treatment

There are signs and symptoms of menopause, which can be eased through intermittent fasting.

Hot Flashes

Hot flashes, also known as vasomotor symptoms, can begin during menopause or when the last menstrual cycle has passed. They usually stay four to five years and are worst after the last menstrual cycle. They continue forever for some women.

Hot flashes are thought to originate inside the hypothalamus, a brain region that regulates body temperature. The thermostat is the middle-aged woman's body, which is unexpectedly adjusted to a lower than average temperature for unsolved reasons. The hot flash seems to a natural cooling response, similar to how a refrigerator starts when the door is opened on a hot day.

For the 15% of women who suffer from the most intense type of hot flashes, they can be particularly distressing. This unfortunate category includes women who have undergone medical menopause or are using tamoxifen to prevent breast cancer. Sweating and pinkish or blistered skin are outward signs of a hot flash, which indicate that a woman's hormone intake is diminishing.

Hot flashes may be accompanied by heart palpitations, nausea, stress, or perhaps a sense of dread; some women report feeling anxious or unsettled just before a hot flash. Hot flashes affect women in various ways—some complain about being too hot or too warm. Many get chills afterward. Night sweats, or hot flashes which happen while sleeping, interrupt sleep, resulting in exhaustion and mood swings.

Treatment of Hot Flashes

Hot flashes are a particularly inconvenient symptom of menopause. They will disturb your relaxation or sleep and cause great discomfort. Although the exact cause of hot flashes remains unknown, they are thought to be due to low estrogen levels and the effect this has on the hypothalamus, the area of the brain that regulates body temperature. Ketone bodies produced during ketosis can help shield and reduce inflammation, as well as regulate body temperature.

Insomnia

Sleep disturbances are a frequent issue for women going through menopause. It's unclear if hot flashes while sleeping trigger sleepiness. Some women claim that they sweat so much that their bed linen becomes wet, and they wake up while others sleep through hot flashes.

According to at least one report, though the woman may not wake up, hot flashes disrupt the most reparative sleep mode. Even if you don't get hot flashes, insomnia can be a concern. Some women may have trouble falling asleep, but it is typical to nap for a few hours, wake up too early, and then be unable to fall asleep again.

It is currently unclear whether sleep disturbances are caused mainly by hormonal changes. As people age, their sleep patterns alter; insomnia is a frequent age-related complaint. Sleep-deprived women may become stressed, agitated, anxious, and cranky as a result. Sleep deficiency is linked to cardiac arrests, including heart failure, so insomnia is not a minor issue.

Treatment of Insomnia

Following IF along with a ketogenic diet during menopause will help you sleep better. Due to the absence of hot sweats, improved blood sugar regulation, a healthy weight, and hormone balance, you will experience good quality sleep. Therefore, now you understand how a ketogenic diet can help ease the symptoms of menopause and improve your overall health, you'll realize the value of implementing it.

Low Sexual Desire

For several reasons, sex drive can wane in middle age. The blood supply to the vagina can be reduced due to lower hormones or age-related shifts in circulation, resulting in a loss of sensation. Intercourse may be rendered uncomfortable by vaginal dryness or thinning.

Women with sleep issues might even be too tired to engage in sex. Urinary incontinence can induce humiliation and can have sex less appealing. Concerns over facial appearance and physical image can also suppress sex desire. Not only might women's sexual response deteriorate as they approach menopause, but also their partners may suffer sexual performance issues.

As a result, women's feelings toward their husbands can be less intense than they previously were. As women approach menopause, their sexual desire, sexual arousal, and rate of intercourse may decrease even further.

Treatment for lack of sexual appetite

Menopause can induce a loss of libido as a result of fluctuating hormones. However, since fat is used to produce sex hormones, a high-fat diet will increase estrogen and testosterone levels, thus boosting the libido.

In studies of a low-fat diet, it was discovered that circulating sex hormones decreased, leading to a reduction in libido. In women, however, research has shown that eating a diet high in fat content improves sexual performance. A high-fat diet with intermittent fasting supplies the body with the natural resources it needs to maintain sex hormone levels, which is crucial for sustaining a healthy menopausal libido.

Depression and mood swings

According to studies, mood variations occur more often during perimenopause, when hormonal changes are the most unpredictable, than throughout the postmenopausal period. Meanwhile, ovarian hormones are stable at a low level. While no clear correlation between decreased estrogen and mood has been identified, mood changes most likely occur as hormonal fluctuations disrupt a woman's daily habits.

These transitions can be overwhelming and make you feel unhappy. Mood fluctuations tend to make you laugh one minute and weep the next, as well as making you feel nervous or sad.

On the other hand, these shifts are generally temporary and do not meet the criteria for diagnosing psychiatric depression, a more severe dysfunctional mental condition. Women experience depression at a higher rate than men. However, there is no proof that low estrogen alone induces psychiatric depression.

While women who have experienced previous bouts of depression are more likely to experience a repetition during menopause, menopause does not induce clinical depression in and of itself. Depression is no more common in postmenopausal women than at any other point in women's lives.

Treatment of Mood Swings

Intermittent fasting with a low-carbohydrate diet can also enhance energy levels. When the body transitions to using fat instead of glucose as its form of nutrition, there will never be any large fluctuations in blood sugar that cause energy levels to drop. Your body now has an almost limitless supply of calories (fat stores) to draw on, allowing it to raise energy levels whenever necessary.

Gaining Weight

Weight gain is a major concern to women during menopause. They may appear to be doing well, but they continue to gain weight. The result is that low estrogen levels cause weight gain, which tends to be concentrated in the abdomen region. This alarms many women who used to have a specific pant size and now have none that fit.

They may have to restrict their calorie intake to lose weight, although this will exacerbate menopausal symptoms. One effect of low-calorie foods is to reduce metabolism. They also hasten the weakening of muscle and bone density, raising the risk of osteoporosis. Muscle and bone loss are inherent during menopause, but why make it worse by eating a low-calorie diet?

Treatment for Weight Gain

When you start to gain weight, the ketogenic diet can be a great way to lose it. A high-fat, low-carbohydrate diet has been proven to help women lose weight and keep it off. In a 2015 study, postmenopausal women who had breast cancer were asked to observe a low-carbohydrate or low-fat diet.

Those who followed a low-carbohydrate diet for six months lost 23.1 pounds, 7.6% of their body mass, and 3.7 inches from their waist. While both parties lost weight, the low-carbohydrate group lost much more. There are several reasons that IF promotes weight loss and enables women in menopause to maintain a healthy weight.

Satiety is improved by increasing protein intake. When you're full and happy, you're less likely to overeat. The elimination of most carbohydrates, on the other hand, results in a reduction in the average calorie intake.

Chapter 3. Popular Ways to Do Intermittent Fasting

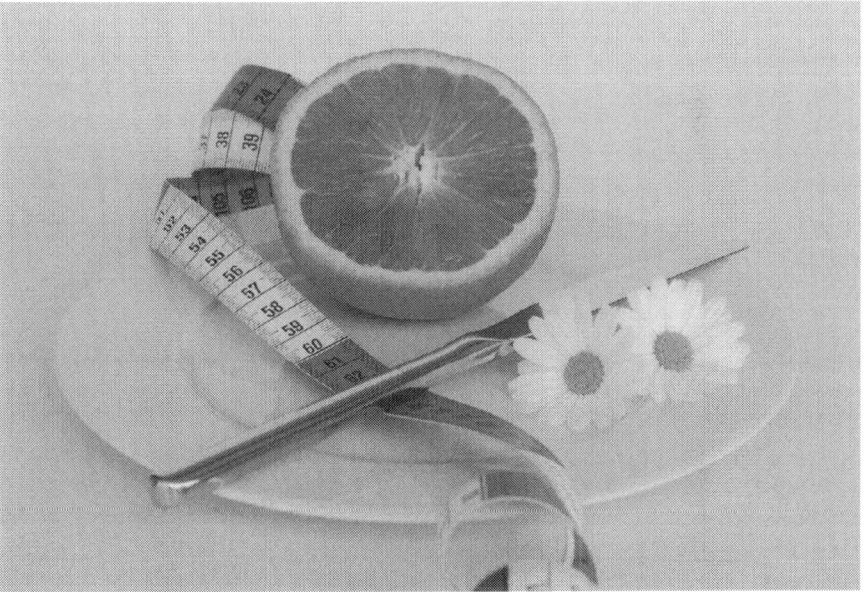

There are several ways you could involve in intermittent fasting. The following types have been proven to give the same effects that have made people start fasting, and some of these benefits include the loss of weight. Some also find that it helps in lowering the risk of getting some diseases.

The 16/8 Method

This includes fasting for a total of 16 hours in the 24 hours of a day. It needs a daily fast of 14 hours for women.

Martin Berkhan, the famous fitness expert, made this method popular. Some refer to it as the Lean gains protocol. It is the most widely known because it is almost natural. The hours you skip meals fall under the time you are either sleeping or working. Most people skip breakfast and finish dinner before eight are doing the 16-hour protocol, but they don't know that.

Women are instructed to fast for 14 to 15 hours because most do better with this short-range, and during the fast, you have to eat healthy foods during the eating window. The results you want to achieve won't be forthcoming if there's a lot of junk in your food.

You can take water and coffee during the fasting hours as well as other drinks that are noncaloric.

To fast with this method, your last meal should be by 8 p.m. while your first meal should be by 12 p.m.

The 5:2 diet

British journalist Michael Mosley popularized this method. It has also been called the fast diet.

This method requires that you limit the number of calories you consume to only 500 for females and 600 for males two days a week. That means you usually eat for five days and reduce the calories in your diet for two days.

For example, you might eat every day of the week except Tuesday and Thursday to reduce the food you consume. You limit the calories for breakfast to 250 for women and 300 for men, while dinner takes the same number of calories.

Eat Stop Eat

This method requires you to do a 24-hour fast either once or twice a week, whichever one is comfortable for you.

An example is not eating from 7 p.m. to 7 p.m. the following day. If you start with dinner on Monday, you don't eat from 7 p.m. Monday to 7 p.m. Tuesday. Do this once or twice a week. If it is once, it should be done mid-week, like Wednesday, and if it is twice, it is good if the days are spread apart, e.g., Monday and Thursday.

You can drink water, coffee, and other noncaloric drinks between fasting periods, but solid foods are not allowed. It is, however, not advisable to start with this method as it requires a lot of energy for long hours without food. Instead, start with 16 hours fasting before plunging into the 24 hours fast.

Alternate-Day Fasting

Most of the health benefits that were revealed are as a result of this method. That is fasting on alternate days.

There are two variations to this method.

•   24-hour full day fasting every other day. This requires you to normally eat for a day and then fast for the next 24 hours.

•   Eating only a few hundred calories. The alternate-day fasting can be very challenging, and this made the experts devise another plan where you only eat a reduced number of calories every other day.

An example is that when you fast on Monday, you normally eat on Tuesday, fast on Wednesday, and continue for the rest of the week.

The Warrior Diet

This method of fasting was made famous by Ori Hofmekler, another fitness expert.

This diet requires you to fast or eat a small or little chunk of food during the day while consuming a huge meal at night, a typical case of fast and feast later. You eat small amounts of fruits and vegetables during the day and fall back to a huge meal.

The meal is best eaten by 4 p.m. After that, no food must be eaten until the following morning when you continue with fruits and vegetables. A feast for dinner and fast for the day.

Spontaneous Meal Skipping

This is a more natural method than the 16/8 because there's no routine. You skip meals when convenient.

This can be done in some instances, such as when you are not hungry or are on a journey and can't find suitable food to eat. You can skip these meals.

There's no routine to this method. You can decide to skip your meal anytime, from lunch to dinner to breakfast. Once you don't follow a routine, you are using this method.

These methods, however, are not suitable for every individual, and you don't need to try everything before you know which is ideal for you.

This guide is for women over 50 years old, and this kind of person often loses energy more rapidly than typical younger youths. Hence, methods, such as the alternate-day fasting and the eat-stop-eat method, are not suitable for women over fifty because these types and processes require a lot of energy, which these women lack.

The 16/8 is not suitable for everyone woman over fifty, but it's a good start if you want to take the fast to another level. There's no magic to it, and no one can tell you what's best for you. You have to discover yourself. Spontaneous meal skipping is a great place to start, but the results won't be as fast as the other methods because of the lack of routine.

The best methods, however, are the eat-stop-eat and the 5:2. These two have routines you can follow, but you don't need to stay away from food. Only consume small calories. This way, you fast with a routine, and the results will be achieved.

Chapter 4.   Getting Started

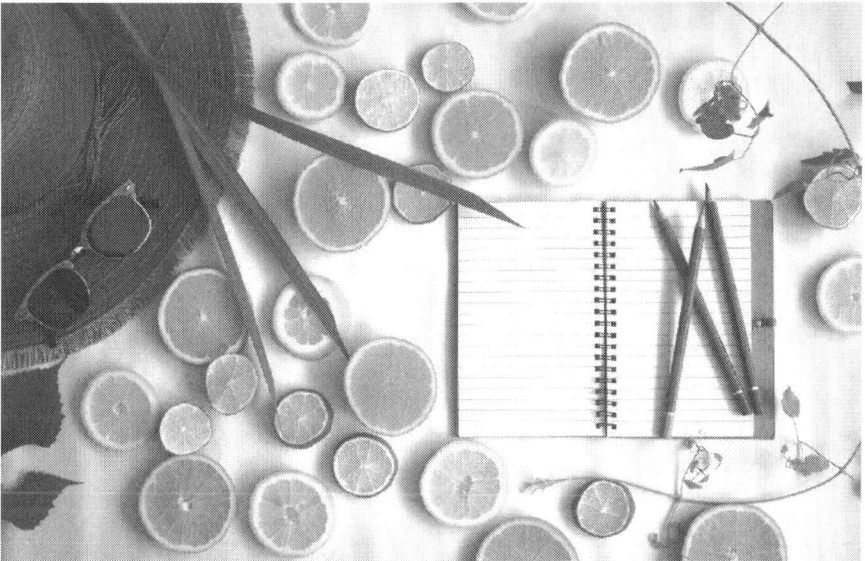

You always have to remember that if you have any medical conditions, please get your doctor's permission before starting any new diet. Changing diets suddenly can cause a woman's hormones to fluctuate, which can cause issues. Pregnant women should also consult a physician; women need to get enough nutrients to support their babies' health. Communicate with your doctor if you have diabetes. If you have any eating disorder, this may not be the diet for you.

Identify Personal Goals

Most of the time, people who start IF have a specific goal in mind. For example, your goal could be to lose weight, work towards getting healthy, or you may want to improve your overall health. Your reason for starting Intermittent fasting will help you choose the eating plan you want to begin.

Pick the Method

You now decide to try out skipping a meal and then try fasting either at 14:10 (14-hour fasting and 10-hour feasting). Another plan you may be able to start is overnight fasting. The majority of the time, you will be asleep with this fasting, making it more manageable. If any of these plans work, you can stay there; if you want more of a challenge, you can continue trying out the other ones.

You have to make sure to choose the one that works best for you. One way to help you choose the best eating plan is to take a look at your lifestyle. Do you get up early and want breakfast as soon as you wake up? If so, make sure to choose a plan that will always have breakfast early. If you are a night owl, you want to start eating later in the day. You will need an eating plan where you can eat from noon-8 or later.

Doing alternate-day fasting is no more effective than doing the 16:8 or 14:10 eating plans. Doing the 24 hours fast is more likely to add to overeating, leading to weight gain. Jama Network did a study that showed that focusing on the number of calories you eat is more beneficial than fasting for 24 hours.

If you are doing alternate day fasting or the 5:2 method, do not fast for two consecutive days. Instead, choose the weekdays to fast instead of the weekends. Weekdays are more structured than the weekends. In addition to having less structure, you will also have more choices in what you eat.

Figure Out Caloric Needs

If you are unsure how to figure out the number of calories and nutrients, you need to consult a dietitian.

Figuring out calories and nutrients is challenging. You can look online to do it, but it's better to ask a dietitian unless you have experience. According to Check Your Health, you can figure out the number of calories you need daily in a few different ways.

The two ways to do this are:

Calculate your basal metabolic rate:

The Basal Metabolic Rate (BMR) determines how many calories you need when you are active versus inactive.

Physical activity - how active you are:

- Do you do light activities a few times a week? An example of this would be a nice walk outside with your pet.
- Do you spend most of your day sitting? If so, you are not active.
- If you do physical activities 2-3 times a week, like speed walking or jogging, you fall into the moderately active category.
- If you work out hard during the week, you fall into the hard exercise category. This is typically into some physical training, such as for a marathon.
- Extra active is for those who train or play professional sports or bodybuilding. Significantly few people fall into this category.

Figure Out A Meal Plan

This is something to remember when choosing which fasting plan is right for you. Do you like to go out for dinner occasionally? Then select the program where you are allocated eating time later in the day.

Is one of your favorite things to do is going out with some friends, having a few drinks, and eating? In this case, you will have to either find something else you can do as a group or do not hang out until your willpower is stronger.

Side Effects

There are a few different side effects that you need to be prepared for. The first few days, it is normal to feel both mentally and physically tired. You get to feel better and have more energy after a week or so.

For the first week, it will be challenging to exercise. This is normal, so do what you can and be easy on yourself. One thing to keep in mind when you plan your workouts while fasting, your body goes into metabolic stress and uses fat instead of sugar for energy.

Foods to Eat and To Avoid

You often hear health experts demonizing sugar and carbohydrates. Now, it should be said that sugar and carbohydrates are not necessarily bad. They become a problem when they are consumed in excess. When you eat too many of these foods, your body has to play catch-up. Naturally, this is where you accumulate fat, gain weight, and see the adverse effects of an unhealthy diet.

So, the intermittent fasting approach calls for you to avoid, or at least significantly reduce, the following foods:

White Starchy Foods

This includes past and potatoes. Starch is metabolized as glucose and immediately goes into fat stores.

Foods Loaded With Carbohydrates

White bread, or anything baked, is usually loaded with a high amount of carbohydrates.

Greasy Foods

Deep-fried and very greasy foods, while tasty, are high in unhealthy fats. These types of fats lead to high cholesterol. These foods are enemy number one for blood vessel health. They generally lead to poor circulation.

Salty Foods

There is nothing wrong with salt unless you eat too much of it. Salting foods to taste is fine. However, excessively salty foods are not only addictive, but they affect your blood pressure and heart health. It is best to switch to sea salt as it contains less sodium.

Sugary Drinks and Alcohol

By "sugary," we mean things like sodas and iced teas. These are loaded with sugar and other chemicals. Also, alcoholic beverages end up accumulating fat in a heartbeat. Now, consuming moderate amounts of alcohol is perfectly fine (1–2 drinks per week). A glass of wine will be great for your heart.

However, excessive alcohol consumption leads to increased fat gains. The reasoning behind this is that alcohol is metabolized by the body the same way sugar is. So, this implies you will be packing extra glucose into your system.

Also, see your doctor see if you have any unknown food allergies. Unfortunately, many folks out there go through their entire lives not knowing they are, in fact, allergic to certain foods. For instance, some folks are lactose intolerant but don't know it.

Other common food allergies are gluten and corn. In particular, corn allergies can lead to quite a bit of digestive distress and inflammation. This is important to note as many of the foods we consume have corn in them.

Chapter 5.   Brunch Recipes

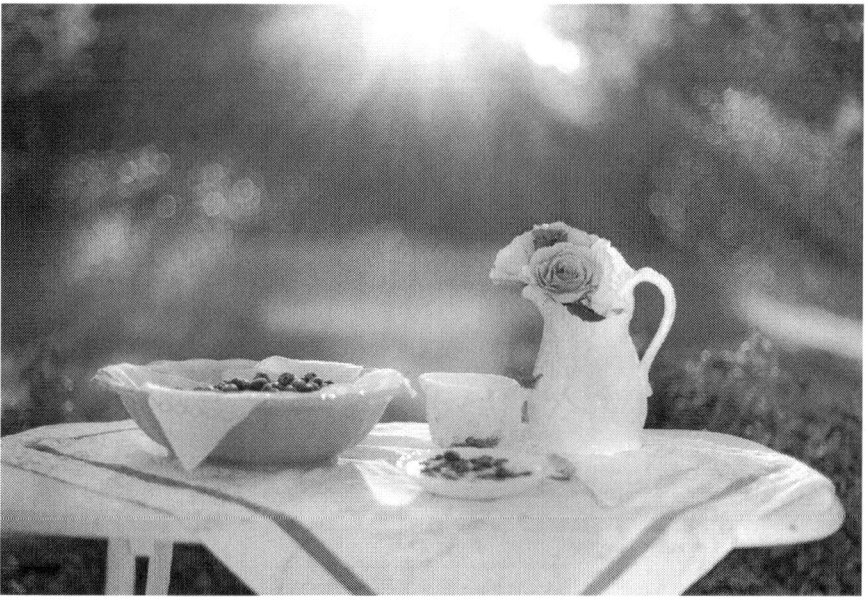

1.   Hot Cross Buns

Preparation Time: 15 minutes
Cooking Time: 30 minutes
Servings: 8
Ingredients:

- Salt (1/2 tsp.)
- Pumpkin spice (1/2 tsp.)
- Cinnamon (1/2 tsp.)
- Ground cloves (1/2 tsp.)
- Coconut flour (1/3 cup)
- Baking powder (1 tsp.)
- Psyllium husks (1/2 cup)
- Swerve granulated sweetener (2 tbsp. or more to taste)
- Eggs (4 medium)
- Boiling water (1 cup)
- Raisins/cacao nibs/chocolate chips
- Powdered sweetener icing mix - keto-friendly (as desired)

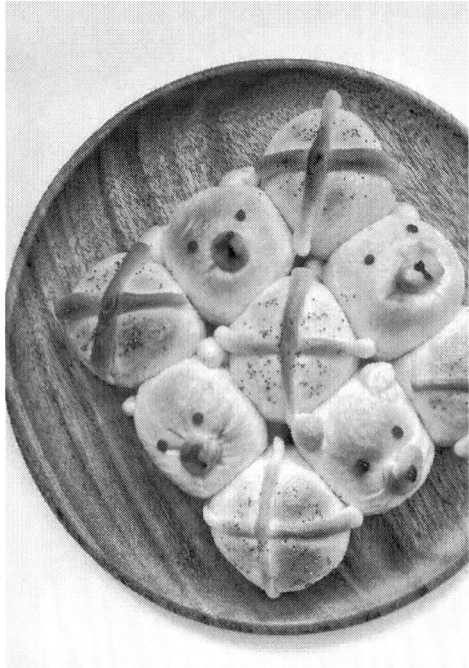

Directions:

1. Whisk each of the dry fixings in a mixing container and fold in the eggs.
2. Put in the boiling water and mix until the mixture is evenly combined.
3. Roll it into eight balls. Add it to a baking pan.
4. Bake them in a fan-assisted oven at 350 F for 20-30 minutes.
5. Prepare the icing. Put plus sign on each hot cross bun using a keto-friendly powdered sweetener confectioners/icing mix and water paste mixture.

Nutrition:
Calories: 84
Fat: 3.1 g
Carbohydrates: 2.1 g
Protein: 5.6 g

2.   Creamy Basil Baked Sausage

Preparation Time: 10 minutes

Cooking Time: 35 minutes

Servings: 12

Ingredients:

- Italian sausage - pork/turkey or chicken (3 lb. or 1.4 kg)
- Cream cheese (8 oz. or 230 g)
- Heavy cream (1/4 cup)
- Basil pesto (1/4 cup)
- Mozzarella (8 oz. or 230 g)

Directions:

1. Set the oven to reach 400 F.
2. Lightly put cooking oil spray to casserole dish. Add the sausage and bake for 1/2 hour.
3. Combine the heavy cream, pesto, and cream cheese.
4. Once done, add the sauce over the casserole and top it off with the cheese.
5. Bake for another ten minutes. The sausage should reach 160 F in the center when checked with a meat thermometer.
6. You can also broil for 3 minutes to brown the cheesy layer.

Nutrition:

Calories: 316

Fat: 23 g

Carbohydrates: 4 g

Protein: 23 g

3. Bacon - Egg and Cheese Cups

Preparation Time:
10 minutes

Cooking Time: 15 minutes

Servings:

Ingredients:

- Bacon (6 strips)
- Large eggs (6)
- Cheese (1/4 cup/25 g)
- Fresh spinach (1 handful)
- Pepper (as desired)

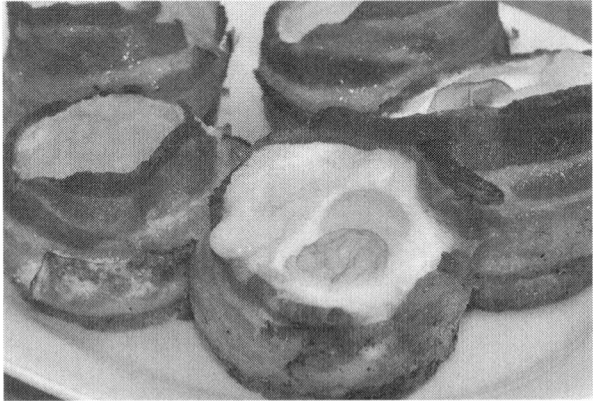

Directions:

1. Set the oven setting to 400 F.
2. Prepare the bacon using medium heat on the stovetop. Place it on towels to drain.
3. Grease six muffin tins with a spritz of oil. Line each tin with a bacon slice, pressing tightly to make a secure well for the eggs.
4. Drain and dry the spinach with a paper towel. Whisk the eggs and combine them with spinach.
5. Add the mixture to the prepared tins and sprinkle with cheese, pepper, and salt.
6. Bake for 15 minutes. Remove when done and serve or cool to store in the fridge.

Nutrition:

Calories: 101

Fat: 7 g

Carbohydrates: 1 g

Protein: 8 g

4.   Baked Avocado Eggs

Preparation Time: 10 minutes

Cooking Time: 15 minutes

Servings: 4

Ingredients:

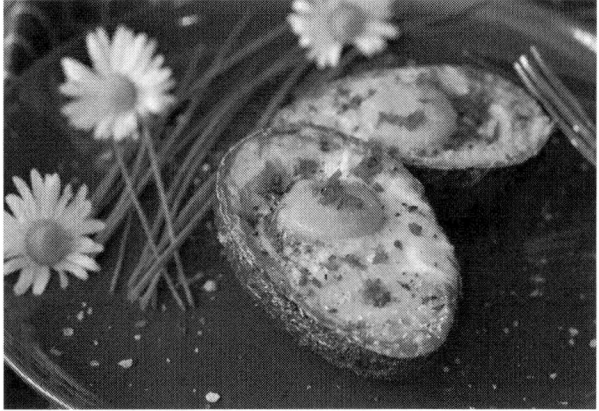

- Avocados (2)
- Black pepper (1 tsp.)
- Parsley - freshly chop (1/4 cup)
- Salt (1/2 tsp.)
- Eggs (4)
- Olive oil (2 tbsp.)

Directions:

1. Heat the oven to 375 F.
2. Wash and dry the avocados, then peel and slice the avocados and remove the pits.
3. Slice a thin edge off the outside of each half to create a flat spot, so they will sit still and not roll.
4. Brush the entire insides of the avocado halves with olive oil.
5. Crack one of the raw eggs into each half of the avocado's center and season the egg with pepper and salt.
6. Bake them for fifteen minutes and sprinkle on the chopped parsley to serve.

Nutrition:

Calories: 260

Fat: 23 g

Protein: 9 g

Carbohydrates: 8 g

5.   Broccoli - Eggs and Sausage with Cheese - Slow-Cooked

Preparation Time: 15 minutes

Cooking Time: 4-5 hours

Servings: 6

Ingredients:

- Medium head of broccoli (1)
- Low-carb sausage links (12. oz./340 g pkg.)
- Shredded cheddar cheese (1 cup - divided)
- Eggs (10)
- Whipping cream (3/4 cup)
- Minced garlic cloves (2)
- Pepper (1/2 tsp.)
- Salt (1/2 tsp.)
- Suggested Size: 6-quart/5.7 L slow cooker

Directions:

1. Chop the broccoli. Mince the garlic and slice the sausage. Grease the pot with some non-stick cooking spray.
2. Layer the broccoli, sausage, and cheese in two-layer segments (6 layers total).
3. Combine the whipping cream, whisked eggs, salt, pepper, and garlic until well mixed. Add to the layered fixings.
4. Secure the lid and cook for two to three hours on high or for 4 to 5 hours on the low setting.
5. It is ready to serve when the edges are browned, and the center is set.

Nutrition:

Calories: 484

Fat: 39 g

Carbohydrates: 4 g

Protein: 26 g

6.   Cheesy Italian Omelet

Preparation Time:
10 minutes

Cooking Time: 10 minutes

Servings: 2

Ingredients:

- Eggs (2)
- Water (1 tbsp.)
- Butter or ghee (1 tbsp.)
- Salami or prosciutto (3 thin slices)
- Basil (6 leaves)
- Mozzarella cheese slices (2 oz. or 56 g)
- Tomato (5 thin slices)
- Salt and black pepper (as desired)

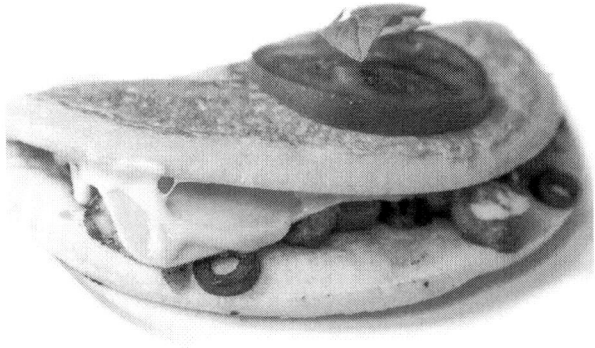

Directions:

1. Whisk the water and eggs in a mixing container.
2. Toss the ghee/butter in a frying pan (medium setting) to melt. Whisk and pour in the eggs and cook for about 30 seconds.
3. Spread out the meat slices over the egg, followed by the cheese, tomatoes, salt, pepper, and basil slices.
4. Cook for approximately two minutes until firm. Flip and continue cooking for another minute before folding in half.
5. Place a top on the skillet to cook using a low-temperature setting.
6. When the center is done, just add the omelet to a plate and serve.

Nutrition:

Calories: 451

Fat: 36 g

Carbohydrates: 3 g

Protein: 33 g

7.   Chicken California Omelet

<u>**Preparation Time:**</u>
10 minutes
<u>**Cooking Time:**</u> 10
minutes
<u>**Servings**</u>: 1
<u>**Ingredients:**</u>

- Bacon (2 slices – cooked and chopped)
- Eggs (2)
- Deli-cut chicken (1 oz./28 g)
- Campari tomato (1)
- Avocado (1/4 of 1)
- Mustard (1 tbsp.)
- Keto-friendly mayo (1 tbsp.)

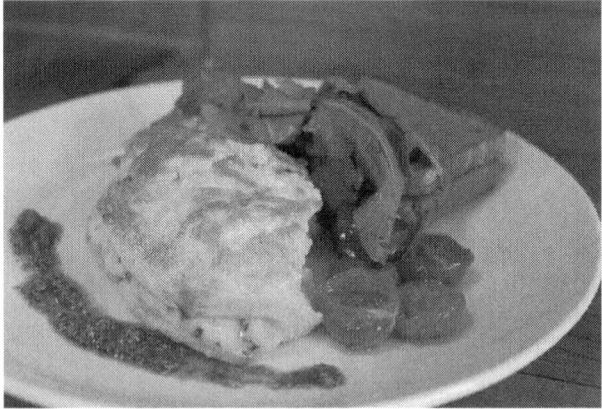

Directions:

1. Beat eggs and add them to a hot skillet.
2. Using the spatula, pull the eggs toward the pan's center to speed up the process and add the pepper and salt.
3. After about five minutes, add the bacon, chicken, avocado, and tomato to the eggs. Squirt the mustard and mayonnaise on one-half.
4. Fold the omelet and cook for five minutes.

Nutrition:

Calories: 308

Fat: 17 g

Carbohydrates: 9.7 g

Protein: 30 g

8.   Cinnamon Breakfast Custard

Preparation Time: 10 minutes
Cooking Time: 50 minutes
Servings: 6
Ingredients:

- Vanilla extract (1 tsp.)
- Heavy cream (2 cups)
- Salt (1/2 tsp.)
- Cinnamon (1 tsp.)
- Egg yolks (2) + whole (2)

Directions:

1. Heat the oven to 300 F.
2. Whisk the cinnamon into the cream. Let it simmer using the low temperature setting until the cream just starts to put off steam. Transfer the pan to a cool burner.
3. Whisk the egg yolks, eggs, and salt.
4. While you are stirring this mixture, continuously pouring in the heavy cream in small amounts and then adding in the vanilla.
5. Pour this mix into a round two-quart baking pan and bake for forty to forty-five minutes.
6. When the cooking time is done, the custard will still be somewhat loose in the center. Serve this dish either warm or cold.

Nutrition:
Calories: 325
Fat: 32.5 g
Carbohydrates: 4.9 g
Protein: 4.6 g

9. Coconut and Walnut Porridge

Preparation Time: 5 minutes

Cooking Time: 5 minutes

Servings: 1

Ingredients:

- Almond butter (1 tbsp.)
- Coconut milk (1/2 cup)
- Crushed walnuts (3 tbsp.)
- Coconut oil (1 tbsp.)
- Cinnamon (1/4 tsp.)
- Desiccated coconut (1 1/2 tbsp.)

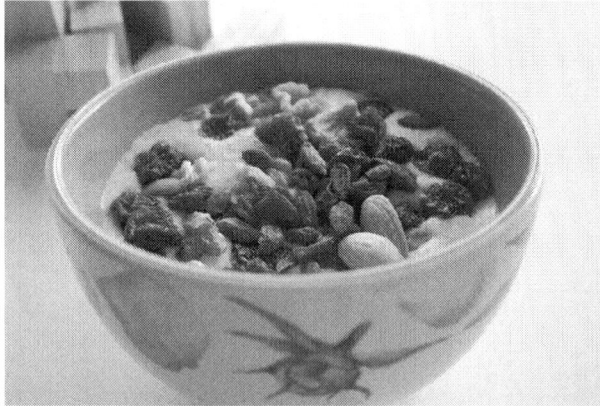

Directions:

1. Warm the coconut oil, milk, and almond butter in a small saucepan.
2. Once it's boiling, mix in the coconut and walnuts.
3. Let it cool for about five minutes and serve.

Nutrition:

Calories: 544

Fat: 65 g

Carbohydrates: 6 g

Protein: 12 g

10.   Cornbread Muffins

Preparation Time: 10 minutes

Cooking Time: 20 minutes

Servings: 6

Ingredients:

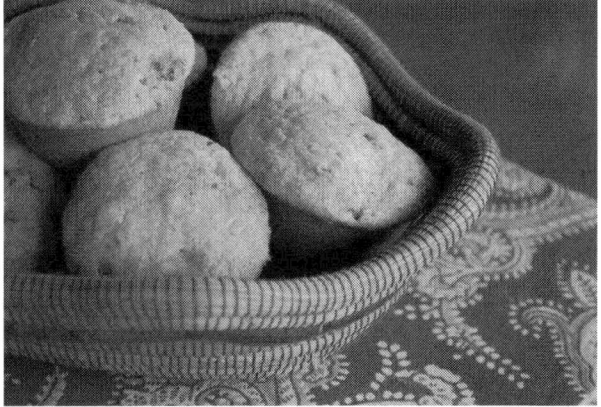

- Almond flour (3/4 cup)
- Coconut flour (1/2 cup)
- Baking powder (2 tsp.)
- Salt (1 tsp.)
- Ghee (2 tbsp.)
- Eggs (3)
- Coconut milk (1/2 cup)

Directions:

1. Set the oven to 350 F.
2. Lightly grease a six-count muffin tin using a spritz of coconut oil or muffin liners.
3. Prepare all the ingredients and mix well in a large bowl.
4. Scoop the batter into the muffin pan.
5. Set the timer for the cornbread to bake for 20 minutes.

Nutrition:

Calories: 191

Fat: 17 g

Carbohydrates: 2 g

Protein: 6 g

11. Garlic Bread

Preparation Time: 15 minutes
Cooking Time: 1 hour
Servings: 20
Ingredients:

- Almond flour (1 1/4 cups)
- Baking powder (2 tsp.)
- Ground psyllium husk powder (5 tbsp.)
- Sea salt (1 tsp.)
- White wine or cider vinegar (2 tsp.)
- Boiling water (1 cup)
- Egg whites (3)

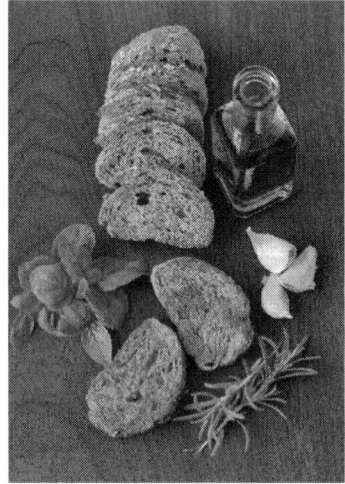

The Garlic Butter:

- Un-chilled butter (4 oz./110 g)
- Garlic (1 clove)
- Fresh parsley (2 tbsp.)
- Salt (1/2 tsp.)

Directions:

1. Set the oven in advance to reach 350° Fahrenheit/177° Celsius.
2. Mince the garlic and finely chop the parsley.
3. Combine the dry fixings in a mixing container.
4. Start a pot of water. Once boiling, pour in the egg whites and vinegar. Whisk using a hand mixer for about 30 seconds.
5. Shape and roll into hot dog-size buns, leaving plenty of space to allow for expansion.
6. Bake using the lower rack for 40-50 minutes. When ready, remove to cool.
7. Prepare the garlic butter and chill.
8. Slice the cooled buns using a serrated knife—spread garlic butter on each half. Reheat the oven to 425 F.
9. Bake until lightly browned (10-15 minutes).

Nutrition:
Calories: 92   Fat: 9 g Carbohydrates: 1 g   Protein: 2 g

12. Sesame Seed Bread

Preparation Time:
1 hour 10 minutes
Cooking Time:
Servings: 6
Ingredients:

- Boiling water (1 cup)
- Sea salt (1/4 tsp)
- Almond flour (1 1/4 cups)
- Baking powder (2 tsp.)
- Sesame seeds (2 tbsp.)
- Psyllium husk powder (5 tbsp.)
- Apple cider vinegar (2 tsp.)
- Egg whites (3)

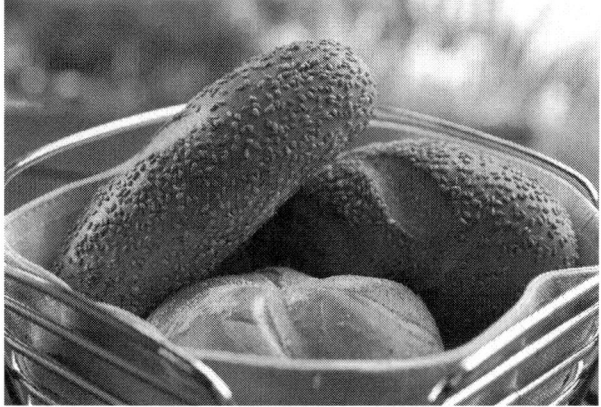

Directions:

1. Program the oven temperature to reach 350 F.
2. Spritz a baking sheet with cooking oil spray. Pour the water into a saucepan to boil.
3. Mix the sea salt, baking powder, almond flour, sesame seeds, and psyllium powder.
4. Pour in the vinegar, hot water, and egg whites. Use a hand mixer (less than 1 minute) to combine.
5. Arrange the bread in the prepared pan.
6. Bake for one hour. Serve and enjoy with a dish of pasta or any time.

Nutrition:
Calories: 100
Fat: 13 g
Carbohydrates: 1 g
Protein: 7 g

13.   Low-Carb Keto Biscuits

Preparation Time: 10 minutes
Cooking Time: 10 minutes
Servings: 9
Ingredients:

- Garlic and onion powder (1/2 tsp. each)
- Almond flour - superfine (1 1/2 cups)
- Baking powder (1 tbsp.)
- Salt (1/4 tsp.)
- Large eggs (2)
- Sour cream/cream cheese/ plain Greek yogurt (1/2 cup)
- Unsalted butter (4 tbsp.)
- Shredded cheddar cheese (1/2 cup)
- Also Needed: 12-cup muffin pan

Directions:

1. Warm the oven to reach 450 F.
2. Lightly grease each of the muffin cavities.
3. Whisk the almond flour with the salt, garlic and onion powder, and baking powder, in a big mixing container.
4. Prepare a small mixing bowl to whisk the sour cream with the eggs and butter. Whisk until the mixture is incorporated and smooth. Thoroughly mix all of the fixings. Fold in the cheese.
5. Scoop batter (1/4 cup) and add it to each muffin mold.
6. Bake the biscuits until the tops are golden (10-11 min.).
7. Allow the biscuits to cool slightly before eating with sausage gravy if desired.

Nutrition:
Calories: 216
Fat: 19 g
Protein: 7 g
Carbohydrates: 3 g

14. Crunchy Zucchini Hash Browns

Preparation Time: 20 minutes
Cooking Time: 20 minutes
Servings: 3
Ingredients:

- 4 medium zucchinis, peeled and grated
- 1 tsp. onion powder
- 1 tsp. garlic powder
- 2 tbsp. almond flour
- 1-1/2 tsp. chili flakes
- Salt and freshly ground pepper to taste
- 2 tsp. olive oil

Directions:

1. Put the grated zucchini in between layers of kitchen towel and squeeze to drain excess water.
2. Pour 1 teaspoon of oil in a pan, preferably non-stick, over medium heat and sauté the potatoes for about 3 minutes.
3. Transfer the zucchini to a shallow bowl and let cool. Sprinkle the zucchini with the remaining ingredients and mix until well combined.
4. Transfer the zucchini mixture to a flat plate and pat it down to make 1 compact layer. Refrigerate and let it sit for 20 minutes.
5. Set your oven to 360 degrees F.
6. Meanwhile, take out the flattened zucchini and divide it into equal portions using a knife or cookie cutter.
7. Lightly brush your air fryer toast oven's basket with the remaining teaspoon of olive oil.
8. Gently place the zucchini pieces into the greased basket and fry for 12-15 minutes, flipping the hash browns halfway through. Enjoy hot!

Nutrition:
Calories: 195
Carbohydrates: 10.4 g
Fats: 13.1 g   Proteins: 9.6 g.

15.　Air Toasted Cheese Sandwich
Preparation Time: 15 minutes
Cooking Time: 20 minutes
Servings: 2
Ingredients:
- 2 eggs
- 4 slices of bread of choice
- 4 slices turkey
- 4 slices ham
- 6 tbsp. half and half cream
- 2 tsp. melted butter
- 4 slices Swiss cheese
- 1/4 tsp. pure vanilla extract
- Powdered sugar and raspberry jam for serving

Directions:
1. Put eggs, vanilla, and cream in a bowl then set aside.
2. Make a sandwich with the bread layered with cheese slice, turkey, ham, cheese slice, and the top slice of bread to make two sandwiches. Gently press on the sandwiches to somewhat flatten them.
3. Spread out kitchen aluminum foil and cut it about the same size as the sandwich and spread the melted butter on the surface of the foil.
4. Soak sandwich in the egg mixture for about 20 seconds on each side.
5. Repeat this for the other sandwich. Place the soaked sandwiches on the directions are foil sheets, then place them on the basket in your fryer or oven.
6. Set on toast and cook for 12 minutes, then flip the sandwiches and brush with the remaining butter and cook for another 5 minutes or until well browned.
7. Place the cooked sandwiched on a plate and top with the powdered sugar and serve with a small bowl of raspberry jam. Enjoy!

Nutrition:
Calories: 346　Carbohydrates: 31.6 g　Fats: 19 g　Proteins: 12 g

16.   Sheet Pan Shakshuka

Preparation Time: 10 minutes
Cooking Time: 10 minutes
Servings: 4
Ingredients:

- 4 large eggs
- 1 large Anaheim chili, chopped
- 2 tbsp. vegetable oil
- 1/2 cup onion, chopped
- 1 tsp. cumin, ground
- 2 minced garlic cloves
- 1/2 cup feta cheese
- 1/2 tsp. paprika
- 1 can of tomatoes
- Salt and pepper

Directions:

1. Sauté the chili and onions in vegetable oil until tender.
2. Pour in the remaining ingredients except for eggs and cook until thick.
3. Make 4 pockets to pour in the eggs.
4. Bake for 10 minutes or 375 F in the oven.
5. Top it off with feta.

Nutrition:

Calories: 320

Fats: 14g

Carbohydrates: 37g

Proteins: 16g

17.   Breakfast Strata

Preparation Time:
2 hours
Cooking Time: 1
hour
Servings: 8
Ingredients:

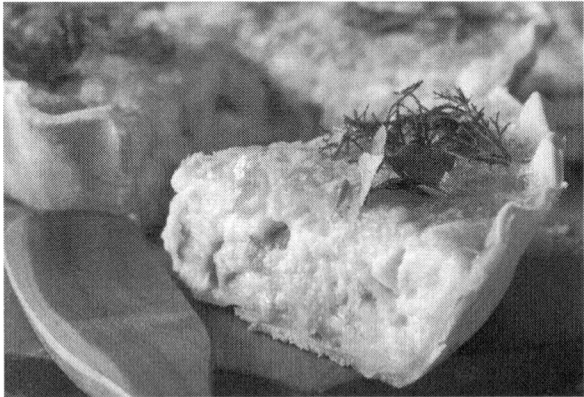

- 18 eggs
- 2 packs of croutons
- 1 pack of cheddar
- Salt and pepper
- 1 pack of chopped spinach
- 3 cups of milk
- 3 cups chopped ham
- 1 jar Red Peppers

Directions:

1. Preheat the oven to 275 F.
2. Spray the pan with a non-stick spray.
3. Spread layers of ham, spinach, cheese, and croutons, and red peppers.
4. Pour eggs mixed with milk and seasoning in the pan and refrigerate for 2 hours.
5. Bake for 1 hour and leave to rest for 15 minutes.

Nutrition:
Calories 140
Fats 5g
Carbohydrates 6g
Proteins 16g

18.   Mini Spinach Quiches

Preparation Time: 10 minutes
Cooking Time: 25 minutes
Servings: 6
Ingredients:

- 2 (9-inch) premade pie crusts, thawed
- 2 eggs
- 1/2 cup sharp cheddar cheese, shredded
- 1/4 cup whole milk
- 1/4 cup heavy cream
- 1/4 cup frozen spinach, drained
- Salt and ground black pepper, to taste

Directions:

1. Arrange the circles into a 6 cups muffin pan.
2. Put holes in the bottom of every pie shell with a fork and put aside.
3. In a bowl, add the remaining ingredients and beat until well combined.
4. Divide the mixture over each pie shell evenly.
5. Turn the oven to line the temperature to 375 degrees F.
6. After preheating, arrange the muffin pan over the roasting rack.
7. When done, remove the muffin pan and put it aside for about 5 minutes before serving.

Nutrition:

Calories: 329
Fats: 22g
Carbohydrates: 23.2g
Proteins: 7.7g

19. Sweet Breakfast Rice

Preparation time: 10 minutes
Cooking time: 5 minutes
Servings: 4
Ingredients:
- 1 1/2 cups almond milk
- 1 1/2 cups cooked brown rice
- 1/2 cup raisins
- 3 ounces shredded coconut
- 1 pear, diced
- 1 apple, diced
- 1 tablespoon maple syrup
- 1 teaspoon cinnamon

Directions:
1. Prepare brown rice.
2. Put and mix all ingredients in a saucepan and heat through.
3. Serve immediately.

Nutrition:
Calories 276
Fats 4g
Carbohydrate 54g
Proteins 6g

20.   Coconut Blackberry Breakfast Bowl

Preparation time: 10 minutes
Cooking time: 5 minutes
Servings: 2
Ingredients:

- 2 tbsp chia seeds
- 1/4 cup coconut flakes
- 1 cup spinach
- 1/4 cup of water
- 3 tbsp ground flaxseed
- 1 cup unsweetened coconut milk
- 1 cup blackberries

Directions:

1. Add blackberries, flaxseed, spinach, and coconut milk into the blender and blend until smooth.
2. Fry coconut flakes in the pan for 1-2 minutes.
3. Pour berry mixture into the serving bowls and sprinkle coconut flakes and chia seeds on top.
4. Serve immediately and enjoy.

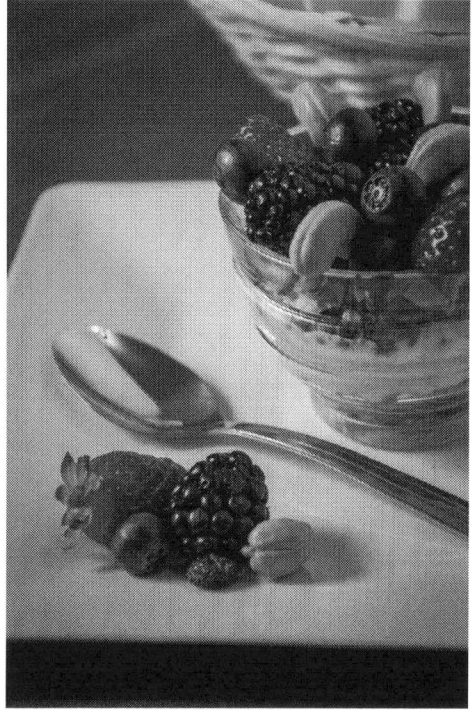

Nutrition:
Calories 182
Fats 11.4 g
Carbohydrates 14.5 g
Proteins 5.3 g

21.   Grain-Free Overnight Oats

Preparation time: 5 minutes + refrigerate overnight

Cooking Time: 0 minute

Servings: 1

Ingredients:

- 2/3 cup unsweetened coconut milk
- 2 tsp chia seeds
- 2 tbsp vanilla proteins powder
- 1/2 tbsp coconut flour
- 3 tbsp hemp hearts

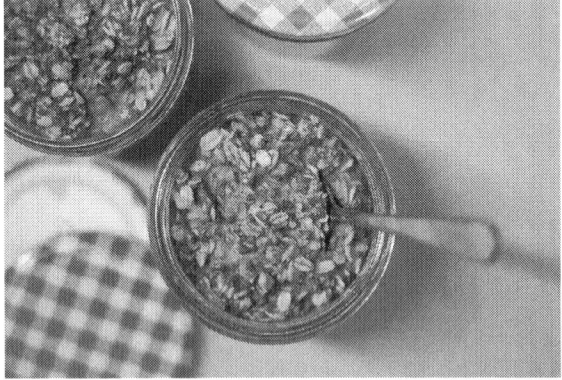

Directions:

1. Add all ingredients into the glass jar and stir to combine—close jar with lid and place in the refrigerator overnight.
2. Top with fresh berries and serve.

Nutrition:

Calories 378

Fats 22.5 g

Carbohydrates 15 g

Proteins 27 g

22.   Broccoli Quiche

Preparation Time:
10 minutes
Cooking Time: 10
minutes
Servings: 1
Ingredients:
- 1 egg
- 1 tbsp
  cheddar
  cheese,
  grated
- 4 broccoli florets
- 3 tbsp heavy cream

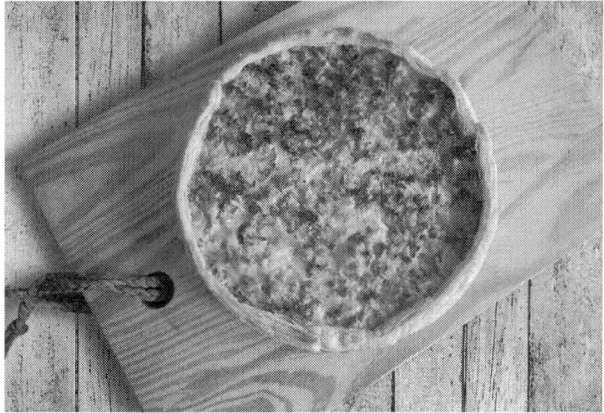

Directions:
1. Spray 5-inch quiche dish with cooking spray.
2. In a bowl, whisk the egg with cheese, cream, pepper, and salt. Add broccoli and stir well.
3. Pour egg mixture into the quiche dish.
4. Place dish into the oven and cook at 325 F for 10 minutes.

Nutrition:
Calories 173
Fats 13 g
Carbohydrates 6.5 g
Proteins 9.9 g

23. Broccoli Fritters

Preparation Time:
10 minutes
Cooking Time: 15
minutes
Servings: 4
Ingredients:

- 3 cups
  broccoli
  florets,
  steam and
  chopped
- 2 cups cheddar cheese, shredded
- 1/4 cup almond flour
- 2 eggs, lightly beaten
- 2 garlic cloves, minced

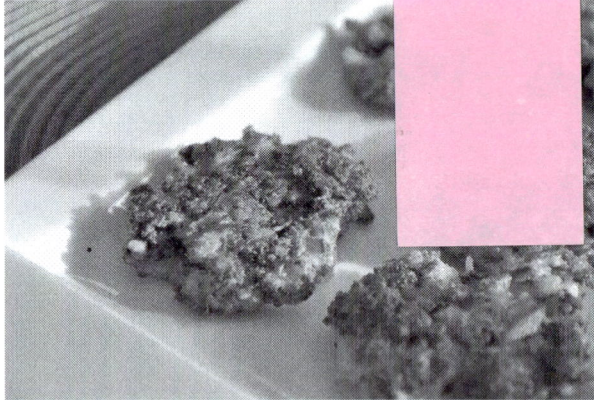

Directions:

1. Line oven with parchment paper.
2. Prepare all ingredients into the mixing bowl and mix until well combined.
3. Make patties from broccoli mixture and place them in the oven.
4. Cook at 375 F for 15 minutes. Turn patties halfway through.

Nutrition:
Calories 128
Fats 4.2 g
Carbohydrates 12 g
Proteins 11 g

24.   Spinach and Ricotta Cups

Preparation Time: 10 minutes
Cooking Time: 10 minutes
Servings: 2
Ingredients:

- 2 large eggs
- 2 tablespoons heavy cream
- 2 tablespoons frozen spinach, thawed
- 4 teaspoons ricotta cheese, crumbled
- Salt and ground black pepper, to taste

Directions:

1. Grease 2 ramekins. In each ramekin, crack one egg.
2. Divide the cream spinach, cheese, salt, and black pepper in each ramekin and gently stir to mix without breaking the yolks.
3. Turn the oven to line the temperature to 330 degrees F.
4. After preheating, arrange the ramekins pan over the roasting rack.
5. Once done cooking, remove the ramekins and place them onto a wire rack to chill for five minutes before serving.

Nutrition:
Calories: 138
Fats 11.4g
Carbohydrates 1.4g
Proteins 7.8g

25.   Radish Hash Browns

Preparation Time: 10 minutes
Cooking Time: 13 minutes
Servings: 2
Ingredients:

- 1 lb. radishes, clean and sliced
- 1 onion, sliced
- 1 tbsp olive oil
- 1 tsp onion powder
- 1 tsp garlic powder
- 1/2 tsp paprika
- 1/4 tsp pepper
- 1/2 tsp salt

Directions:

1. Toss the sliced radishes and onion with olive oil.
2. Spray oven with cooking spray.
3. Spray radish and onion mixture into the oven and cook at 360 F for 8 minutes.
4. Transfer radish and onion mixture into the mixing bowl. Add onion powder, garlic powder, paprika, pepper, and salt and toss well.
5. Return radish and onion mixture into the oven and cook for 5 minutes more.
6. Serve and enjoy.

Nutrition:

Calories 125
Fats 7.4 g
Carbohydrates 13.6 g
Proteins 3.6 g

Chapter 6.   Lunch Recipes

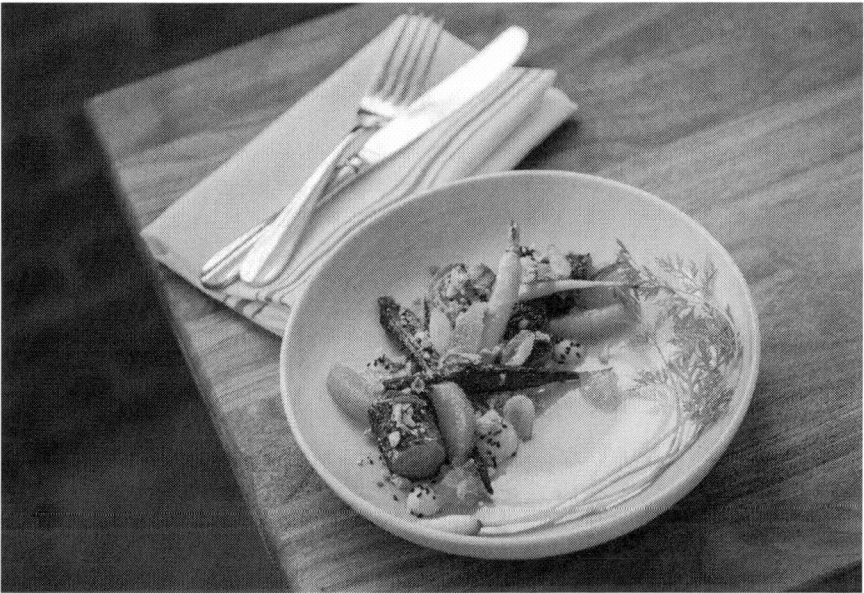

26.   Camembert Mushrooms

Preparation Time: 5 minutes
Cooking Time: 15 minutes
Servings: 3
Ingredients:
- 2 tbsp. butter
- 4 oz. Camembert cheese, diced
- 2 tsp. garlic, minced
- 1 lb. button mushroom, halved
- Black pepper to taste

Directions:
1. Place a skillet over medium-high heat. Add the butter and let it melt.
2. Once melted, add the garlic and sauté until translucent; it should take 3 minutes.
3. Add the mushrooms and cook for 10 minutes.
4. Season with pepper and serve. Enjoy!

Nutrition:
Calories: 161
Fats: 13 g
Carbohydrates: 3 g
Protein: 9 g

27 The Best Garlic Cilantro Salmon

Preparation Time: 10

Cooking Time: 15 minutes

Se ...

In ...

- ... mon filet
- 1 tbsp. butter
- 1 lemon
- 1/4 cup fresh cilantro leaves, chopped
- 4 garlic cloves, minced
- 1/2 tsp. kosher salt
- 1/2 tsp. black pepper, freshly ground

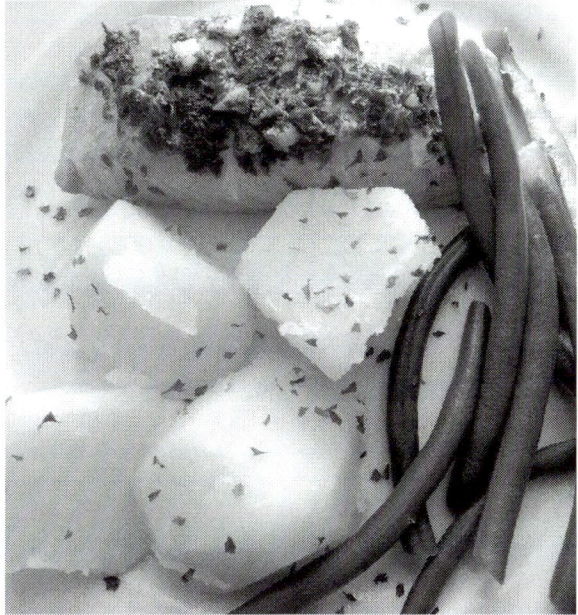

Directions:

1. Preheat the oven to 400 F.
2. On a baking sheet, place the salmon fillet skin-side down.
3. Squeeze the lemon over the salmon.
4. Season the salmon with cilantro and garlic, pepper, and salt.
5. Slice the butter thinly and place pieces evenly over the salmon.
6. Bake for about 7 minutes, depending on thickness.
7. Set the oven to broil and cook 5–7 minutes, or until the top is crispy.
8. Remove the salmon from the oven and serve immediately.

Nutrition:

Calories: 140

Carbohydrates: 3.5 g

Fats: 4 g

Protein: 24.9 g

28.　Crispy Oven Roasted Salmon

Preparation Time: 5 minutes
Cooking Time: 20 minutes
Servings: 3
Ingredients:

- 1 lb. salmon fillet
- 1/4 tsp. sea salt
- 2 tbsps. coconut oil
- 1/2 tsp. mixed herbs (thyme, oregano, marjoram)

Directions:

1. Prepare oven to 425 F.
2. Arrange baking sheet with parchment paper and grease with 1 tablespoon of coconut oil.
3. Place the salmon fillet on the lined baking sheet skin-side down.
4. Season with salt and herbs.
5. Place 1 tablespoon of coconut oil on top of the salmon.
6. Cook until your desired level of crispiness is reached. Serve.
7. You can store the dish in a glass container in the fridge for up to 2 days.

Nutrition:

Calories: 400
Carbohydrates: 0.2 g
Fats: 28.7 g
Protein: 35.8 g

29.   Baked Garlic Ghee Chicken Breast

Preparation Time: 5 minutes
Cooking Time: 30 minutes
Servings: 1
Ingredients:
- 1 chicken breast
- 1 tsp. garlic powder
- 1 tbsp. ghee
- 2 garlic cloves, chopped
- 1 tsp. sea salt
- 1 tsp. chives, diced

Directions:
1. Preheat oven to 350 F.
2. Place the chicken breast on a piece of foil.
3. Season with sea salt, garlic powder, chopped fresh garlic.
4. Top with the ghee and rub everything into the chicken breast.
5. Wrap the chicken breast in the foil and place it on a baking tray.
6. Bake for 30 minutes, or until chicken breast is cooked through, with a meat thermometer reading above 165 F.
7. Serve with more salt and ghee to taste. Cut the chicken breast into slices and sprinkle the diced chives on top.

Nutrition:
Calories: 264
Carbohydrates: 6.1 g
Fats: 15.5 g
Protein: 23.7 g

30.   Lemon Baked Salmon

Preparation Time:
5 minutes
Cooking Time: 20
minutes
Servings: 2
Ingredients:

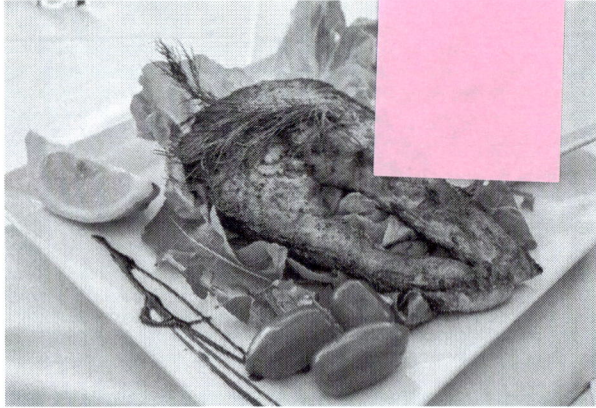

- 12 oz. salmon fillets
- 2 lemons, sliced thinly
- 2 tbsps. olive oil
- Salt and black pepper, to taste
- 3 sprigs thyme

Directions:

1. Preheat the oven to 350 F.
2. Place half the sliced lemons on the bottom of a baking dish.
3. Place the salmon fillets over the lemons and cover with the remaining lemon slices and thyme.
4. Drizzle olive oil over the dish and cook for 20 minutes.
5. Season with salt and pepper.

Nutrition:
Calories: 571
Carbohydrates: 2 g
Fats: 44 g
Protein: 42 g

31.   Chicken and Prosciutto Spiedini

Preparation Time: 15 minutes
Cooking Time: 10 minutes
Servings: 8
Ingredients:

- 8 raw chicken tenders
- 8 oz. block provolone cheese
- 8 slices prosciutto
- 1/2 tsp. kosher salt
- 1/8 tsp. ground black pepper
- 16 fresh basil leaves
- 1/4 tsp. garlic powder
- 8 skewers

Directions:

1. Combine the garlic powder, kosher salt, and pepper.
2. Cut the chicken tenders off the tendons, cutting them into 1/2-inch pieces.
3. Season the chicken with the spice mixture.
4. Cut the provolone cheese into pieces about 1-2 inches long.
5. On a cutting board, place a slice of prosciutto. Then top with 1 chicken tender and 2 leaves of fresh basil. Place 1 piece of cheese across the basil.
6. Carefully roll the bundle and skewer it.
7. Preheat a grill to 325–375 F. Grill for about 3–5 minutes per side, or until a thermometer reads 165 F in the center and the skewers are cooked through. Serve warm.

Nutrition:
Calories: 174
Carbohydrates: 0.75 g
Fats: 10 g
Protein: 20 g

32.   Pimiento Cheese Meatballs

Preparation Time:
30 minutes
Cooking Time: 20
minutes
Servings: 4
Ingredients:

- 1/3 cup mayonnaise
- 1/4 cup pimientos or pickled jalapeños
- 1 tsp. chili or paprika powder
- 1 tbsp. Dijon mustard
- 1 pinch cayenne pepper
- 4 oz. grated cheddar cheese
- For the Meatballs:
- 1 1/2 lb. ground beef
- 1 egg
- 2 tbsps. butter for frying
- Salt and pepper

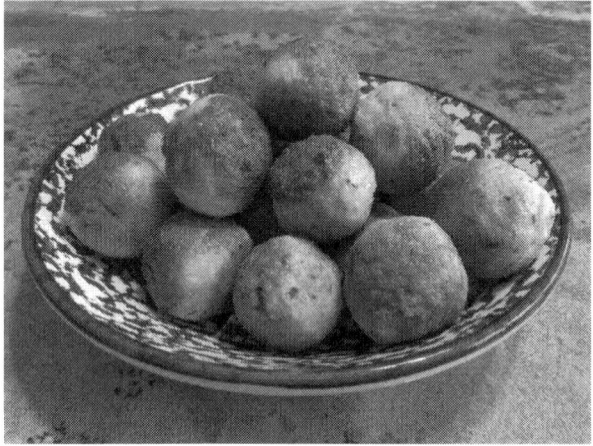

Directions:

1. Prepare all the ingredients in a bowl for the pimiento cheese. Then, add the egg and some ground beef to the cheese mixture.
2. To mix the ingredients, you may need a wooden spoon or use your hands. We recommend using latex gloves when handling raw meat.
3. Add salt and pepper to taste. Once you've used the mixture to form large meatballs, fry them in butter in a pan over medium heat until they are cooked thoroughly.
4. Serve it with a green salad and homemade mayonnaise.

Nutrition:
Calories: 660
Fats: 53 g
Carbohydrates: 1 g   Protein: 42 g

33.   Asian Chicken Wings

Preparation Time:
10 minutes

Cooking Time: 35
minutes

Servings: 5

Ingredients:

- 2 lbs. chicken wings
- 2 tbsps. sesame oil
- 1/4 cup tamari sauce
- 1 tbsp. ginger powder
- 2 tsp. white wine vinegar
- 3 garlic cloves, minced
- 1/4 tsp. sea salt

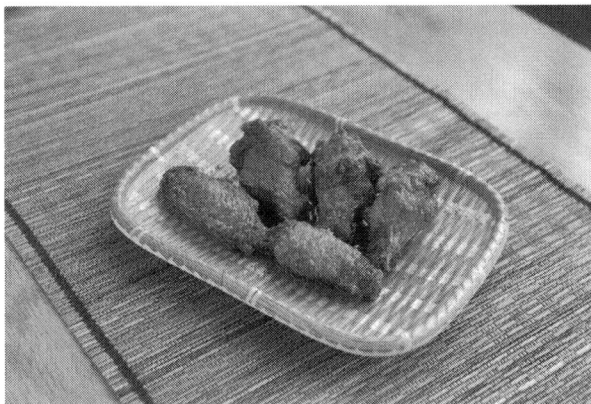

Directions:

1. Preheat oven to 400 F.
2. In a large container, beat together the ginger powder, sesame oil, salt, tamari sauce, vinegar, and garlic.
3. Add the wings to the mixture and stir to coat.
4. Place the wings on a lined baking sheet and bake for 30–35 minutes until golden and crispy.
5. If you want it crispier, turn on the broiler for a few minutes. Enjoy!

Nutrition:

Calories: 277

Carbohydrates: 1 g

Fats: 22 g

Protein: 18 g

34.   Bok Choy Samba

Preparation Time: 5 minutes
Cooking Time: 15 minutes
Servings: 3
Ingredients:
- 1 onion sliced
- 4 bok choy, sliced
- 4 tbsps. coconut cream
- Salt and ground black pepper, to taste
- 1/2 cup parmesan cheese, grated

Directions:
1. Start by tossing the bok choy with salt and black pepper for seasoning.
2. Add oil to any large-sized pan and sauté the onion in it for 5 minutes.
3. Stir in the bok choy and coconut cream. Stir-cook for 6 minutes.
4. Toss in the cheese and cover the skillet to cook over low heat for 3 minutes. Enjoy fresh and warm.

Nutrition:
Calories: 112
Fats: 4.9 g
Carbohydrates: 1.9 g
Protein: 3 g

35. Bacon-Wrapped Salmon

Preparation Time: 10 minutes

Cooking Time: 20 minutes

Servings: 2

Ingredients:

- 2 salmon fillets
- 1 tbsp. olive oil
- 4 slices bacon
- Lemon wedges
- 2 tbsps. tarragon

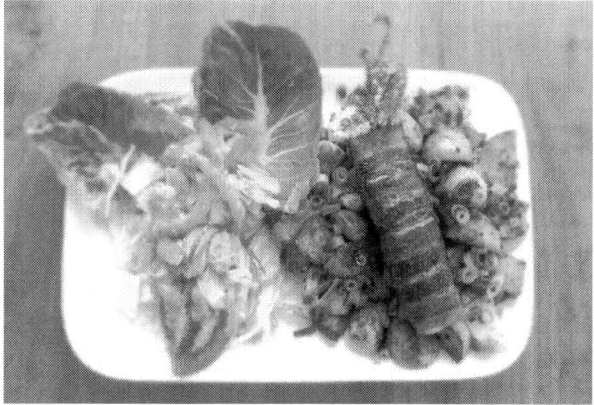

Directions:

1. Preheat the oven to 350 F.
2. Pat the fillets dry.
3. Wrap the bacon around the salmon fillets.
4. Place fillets on a roasting tray and drizzle with olive oil.
5. Bake for 15–20 minutes.
6. Garnish with lemon wedges and chopped tarragon.

Nutrition:

Calories: 612

Carbohydrates: 7.1 g

Fats: 42 g

Protein: 53.3 g

36.   Aromatic Dover Sole Fillets

Preparation Time: 5 minutes

Cooking Time: 20 minutes

Servings: 2

Ingredients:

- 6 Dover sole fillets
- 1/4 cup virgin olive oil
- 1 lemon zested
- A dash of cardamom powder
- 1 cup fresh cilantro leaves
- Pinch of sea salt

Directions:

1. Bring the fillets to room temperature.
2. Set the oven's broiler to high.
3. Pour half of the oil into an oven tray.
4. Put half of the lemon zest, cilantro leaves, and cardamom powder.
5. Arrange fillets in the mixture and put the remaining ingredients.
6. Set under the broiler for about 7–8 minutes, or until the fish breaks easily with a fork and is not transparent. Serve immediately.

Nutrition:

Calories: 244

Carbohydrates: 2.9 g

Fats: 17.9 g

Protein: 18.6 g

37.　Pinchos de Pollo Marinated Grilled Chicken Kebabs

Preparation Time: 15 minutes (+2 hours)

Cooking Time: 10 minutes

Servings: 4

Ingredients:

- 1 1/2 lb. skinless chicken breast (boneless)
- 1 tbsp. minced garlic
- 1/2 tsp. Himalayan salt, fine
- 1/2 tsp. freshly ground black pepper
- 1 tsp. dried oregano
- 1 tbsp. extra-virgin olive oil
- 1 lime juiced
- 7–9 skewers

Directions:

1. Have ready 7–9 soaked skewers.
2. Combine the salt, garlic, pepper, lime juice, oregano, and oil in a bowl.
3. Cut the chicken breast into 1-inch chunks and place it in a container with a lid.
4. Put marinade over the chicken and stir. Place cover and refrigerate for 2 hours or overnight.
5. Preheat a grill to 325–375 F.
6. Remove the chicken from the refrigerator and thread it onto the skewers, leaving a very small space between each piece and spreading it as flat as possible.
7. Once the grill is hot, grill the kebabs over direct medium heat, about 8–10 minutes total, keeping the lid closed until the chicken is no longer pink in the center and is firm to the touch, turning once or twice during cooking. Take care not to overcook.
8. Remove from the grill and serve immediately!

Nutrition:

Calories: 290

Carbohydrates: 3 g

Fats: 10 g Protein: 9 g

38. Mediterranean Stuffed Chicken

Preparation Time: 35 minutes

Cooking Time: 25 minutes

Servings: 2

Ingredients:

- 2 skinless and boneless chicken breast halves
- 1/4 cup feta cheese, crumbled
- 2 tbsp. red sweet peppers, finely chopped, roasted
- 15 oz. bell peppers, roasted
- 2 tbsp. green onion, thinly sliced
- 2 tbsp. snipped fresh oregano
- 1/2 tsp. oregano, crushed, dried
- 1/2 tsp. black pepper, ground

Directions:

1. In each chicken breast, cut a pocket, usually in the thickest part, then put the chicken breast aside.
2. Take a bowl and mix it with the feta cheese, roasted peppers, oregano, and green onion.
3. Fill the pockets of the chicken breasts with the mixture you now have.
4. Place the chicken breast into a frying pan and let them cook over medium heat.
5. When cooked, the chicken breast will turn white (from pink), and the temperature of the thickest part should be around 170 F. As an alternative, you can use a grill, but the instructions are still the same.
6. After around 15 minutes over medium heat, you will need to flip over the chicken breasts (halfway through) and let them grill for 10 more minutes.
7. Put the chicken aside and let it cool. We recommend veggies as a side dish, but it's your call if you feel like using rice or potatoes.

Nutrition:

Calories: 186

Fats: 8.6 g

Carbohydrates: 1.5 g

Protein: 23.4 g

39. Cheesy Pottery Zucchini

Preparation Time: 10 minutes
Cooking Time: 50 minutes
Servings: 4
Ingredients:
- Non-stick cooking spray
- 2 cups of zucchini
- 2 tablespoons leeks thinly diced
- 1/2 teaspoon of salt
- Freshly ground black pepper
- 1/2 teaspoon of dried basil
- 1/2 tablespoon of dried oregano
- 1/2 cup of cheddar cheese, grated
- A quarter cup of heavy cream
- 4 tablespoons of parmesan cheese
- 1 tablespoon of butter

Directions:
1. Prepare oven to 370 F. Grease a saucepan gently. Use a non-stick mist for cooking.
2. Add one tablespoon of new garlic, hazelnuts. Place 1 cup of zucchini slices in the dish; add one spoonful of leeks; sprinkle.
3. Season with oil, basil, pepper, and oregano. Finish Cheddar cheese with 1/4 cup. Echo the layers once again.
4. Whisk the heavy cream in a mixing dish with Parmesan, butter, and garlic. Put this over the layer of zucchini and the layers of cheese.
5. Position in the preheated furnace and cook to the outside for around 40 to 45 minutes till the edges are beautifully browned. Spray with chopped chives, if required.

Nutrition:
Calories: 214
Fat: 11.7g
Carbohydrates: 9g
Protein: 12.9g

40.   Quick Steak Salad

Preparation Time: 5 minutes

Cooking Time: 20 minutes

Servings: 4

Ingredients:

- 4 tablespoons of olive oil
- 16- ounces flank steak, flavored with salt and pepper
- 2 Cucumbers
- 1 cup of sliced carrots
- 2 ripe avocadoes finely sliced, peeled, and trimmed
- 4 Small-sized heirloom tomatoes
- 4 ounces of sliced arugula
- 2 tablespoons of clean baby coriander
- Six spoons of lime juice

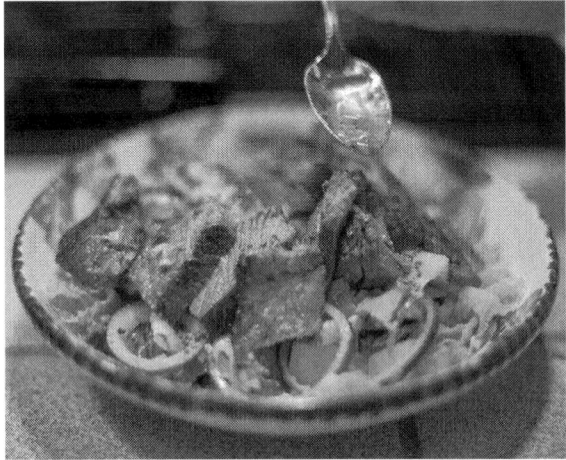

Directions:

1. Heat 1 spoonful of olive oil over medium to high heat in a cup.
2. Prepare the sides Steak, turn once or twice, for 5 minutes. Let it stay for 10 minutes, so finely slice over the grain. Place the meat over to one pot.
3. Include cucumbers, shallots, avocado, tomatoes, fresh coriander, and baby arugula.
4. Sprinkle the salad with lime juice and the remaining one tablespoon of olive oil.
5. Serve cooled sufficiently and serve!

Nutrition:

Calories: 200

Fat: 17.4g

Carbohydrates: 0.7g

Protein: 24.9g

41.   Mushrooms Stuffed with Beef and Goat Cheese

Preparation Time: 5 minutes

Cooking Time: 20 minutes

Servings: 4

Ingredients:

- 8- ounces of ground beef
- 4- ounces of ground pork
- Kosher salt and black pepper
- 1 cup of goat cheese
- 4 tablespoons of Romano cheese crumbled, grated
- 4 spoonsful of shallot, diced
- 2 garlic cloves, dry
- 2 teaspoons of oregano dried basil
- 1 teaspoon of rosemary dry
- 40- button Champignons, stems cut

Directions:

1. Add all ingredients in a baking pot, except perhaps the mushrooms.
2. Then stuff the mushrooms with the filling.
3. Bake for about 18 minutes in the oven and bake at 370 F. Service warm and cold.

Nutrition:

Calories: 222

Fat: 19.2g

Carbohydrates: 3g

Protein: 28.6g

42.   Saucy Steak Skirt with Broccoli

Preparation Time: 2 hours

Cooking Time: 25 minutes

Servings: 4

Ingredients:

- 2 pounds skirt steak
- 2 tablespoons of butter cut into parts, room temperature
- 2 pounds of broccoli
- 2 cups of scallions sliced into florets
- 4 cloves of garlic sliced to bits

For marinade

- 2 teaspoons of black pepper
- 4 teaspoons of red pepper
- 2 teaspoons of sea salt flakes
- 2 tablespoons of olive oil
- 1 tablespoon of tamari sauce
- 1 cup of Vinegar wine

Directions:

1. Ingredients for the marinade are carefully mixed in a ceramic pot.
2. Add the beef and allow it to remain in your fridge for 2 hours.
3. Dissolve one spoonful of butter over strong to medium-high heat in a pan.
4. Cook the dishes broccoli, regularly mixing for 2 minutes, till soft yet bright green, reserve.
5. Melt the remaining butter tablespoon into the skillet—Cook the once warm, scallions and garlic for about 2 minutes, before aromatic, reserve.
6. Then grill the steak, applying a limited amount of marinade.
7. Process till smooth brown on both levels, perhaps 10 minutes and so.
8. Insert the stored vegetables and start cooking for several minutes or until everything is ready and heated.

Nutrition:

Calories: 264   Fat: 20g

Carbohydrates: 2.1g   Protein: 18.9g

43.   Skillet Chinese Ground Beef

Preparation Time: 10 minutes

Cooking Time: 20 minutes

Servings: 4

Ingredients:

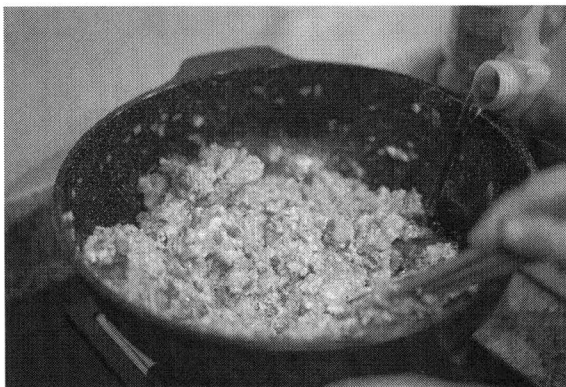

- 2 tablespoons of sesame oil
- 1-pound chuck
- 2 shallots
- 2 chopped garlic cloves
- Some cloves
- 2 (1/2) "slice of ginger root, peeled and rubbed
- 2 bell peppers
- 8 ounces of brown mushrooms crushed and diced
- 2 tablespoons of tamari soy
- 2 tablespoons of rice wine
- 4-star anise
- Himalayan salt and black pepper, to taste

Directions:

1. Put oil in the saucepan over a medium flame. Then roast the ground chuck until it's cooked or isn't pink anymore, reserve.
2. Then in pan drippings, cook the shallot, garlic, ginger, pepper, and mushrooms.
3. Finally, apply the rest of the ingredients and the retained beef to the saucepan.
4. Decrease temperature to medium-low; allow it to simmer for 2 to 3 more minutes. Then serve.

Nutrition:

Calories: 242

Fat: 24g

Carbohydrates: 6g

Protein: 26.9g

44.   Chicken Breasts Ranch with Cheese

Preparation Time: 5 minutes
Cooking Time: 20 minutes
Servings: 4
Ingredients:

- 4 Chicken breasts
- 4 spoons of sugar
- 2 tablespoons of salt
- 1 teaspoon of Garlic
- 1 teaspoon of cayenne pepper paste
- 1 teaspoon of black peppercorns, ground
- 1 teaspoon ranch seasoning blend
- 8 ounces of Ricotta cheese
- 1 cup of Monterey-Jack cheese
- 8 slices of bacon
- 1/2 cup of minced scallions

Directions:

1. Preheat your oven to 370 F. Sprinkle with melted butter over the chicken.
2. Flavor chicken with salt and garlic powder, a seasoning blend of cayenne pepper, black pepper, and ranch.
3. Set moderate heat a cast-iron skillet. Boil the chicken for 3 to 5 minutes by hand.
4. Place the chicken in a lightly greased baking dish. Add bacon and cheese.
5. Bake for 12 minutes. Scallions on end right before serving.

Nutrition:
Calories: 295
Fat: 3g
Carbohydrates: 2g
Protein: 19g

45.   Chicken Unique Salad

Preparation Time: 10 minutes

Cooking Time: 20 minutes + 1-hour refrigerate

Servings: 4

Ingredients:

- 2 skinless chicken breasts
- 1/2 cup mayonnaise
- 1/2 cup of sour cream
- 4 spoons Cottage cheese, ambient temperature
- Salt and black pepper as per taste
- 1/2 cup of Sunflower seeds
- 1 avocado
- 1/2 tablespoons of peeled and cubed garlic
- 4 spoonsful of sliced scallions

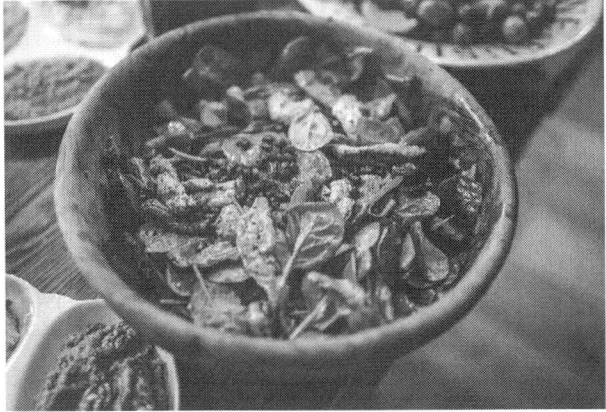

Directions:

1. Place a very well-salted pot of water to a gentle simmer.
2. Place the chicken in hot water; turn the heat down low, and let the chicken stay for 15 minutes.
3. Remove the bowl, then; cut the chicken into pieces of bite-size.
4. Add the rest of the ingredients and mix them properly. Keep in the fridge for an hour.

Nutrition:

Calories: 284

Fat: 19g

Carbohydrates: 3g

Protein: 17.6g

46.   Chicken Quesadilla Chaffle

Preparation Time: 10 minutes
Cooking Time: 15 minutes
Servings: 4
Ingredients:

- 1 teaspoon of taco seasoning
- 1 cup of cooked and chopped chicken
- 2 beaten eggs
- 1 cup of finely grated cheddar cheese

Directions:

1. Preheat the waffle iron.
2. In a medium bowl, mix the eggs, taco seasoning, and cheddar cheese. Add the chicken and combine well.
3. Open the iron, lightly oil with cooking spray, and pour in 1/2 of the mixture.
4. Close the iron and cook until brown and crispy, 7 minutes.
5. Remove the Chaffle onto a plate and set it aside.
6. Make another Chaffle using the remaining mixture. Serve afterward.

Nutrition:

Calories: 135
Fat: 10g
Carbohydrates: 1g
Protein: 11g

47.   Chaffle and Chicken Lunch Plate

Preparation Time: 10 minutes
Cooking Time: 15 minutes
Servings: 4
Ingredients:

- A pinch salt
- 1 cup of shredded jack cheese
- 2 large egg
- Salt
- 2 teaspoons of garlic paste
- 2 teaspoons of avocado oil
- 2 chicken legs
- Pepper to taste
- 2 egg

Directions:

1. Heat your square waffle-making machine and oil with cooking spray.
2. Pour Chaffle batter into the skillet and cook for about 3 minutes.
3. Put a pan over medium heat and heat the oil.
4. Once the oil is hot, add chicken thigh and garlic then, cook for about 5 minutes.
5. Flip and cook for another 3-4 minutes. Season with pepper and salt and mix well—Transfer cooked thigh to plate.
6. Fry the egg in the same pan for about 1-2 minutes.
7. Once Chaffle are cooked, serve with a fried egg and chicken thigh. Enjoy!

Nutrition:
Calories: 156
Fat: 9g
Carbohydrates: 3g
Protein: 17g

48.   Sausage Ball Chaffle

Preparation Time: 5 minutes
Cooking Time: 10 minutes
Servings: 4
Ingredients:
- 4 tablespoons of flour
- 1 cup of grated cheddar cheese
- 2 eggs
- 1 pound of Italian sausage
- 2 teaspoons of baking powder
- 1/2 cup of grated parmesan cheese

Directions:
1. In a bowl, combine Italian sausage, flour, baking powder, cheddar cheese, and egg. Make sure you
2. kneed these ingredients well.
3. Then turn on the waffle-making machine and preheat it to medium heat.
4. Then sprinkle some parmesan cheese on the waffle-making machine and let it cook for about 30 seconds.
5. Add the mixture on top of the cheese and close the lid of the waffle machine.
6. Let the Chaffle cook for about 3 to 5 minutes until it is golden brown.

Nutrition:
Calories: 245
Fat: 13.4 g
Protein: 19.2 g
Carbohydrates: 1.1 g

49.   Simple Curry Turkey

Preparation Time: 10 minutes
Cooking Time: 50 minutes
Servings: 4
Ingredients:
- 3 teaspoons of Sesame oil
- 1 pound of turkey legs
- 2 cloves
- 1 red chili pepper
- 1/2 tablespoon of minced garlic
- 1/2 teaspoon of ginger powder
- 1/4 Turmeric powder
- 1 teaspoon of red curry paste
- 1 cup of unsweetened coconut milk
- 1/2 cup of water
- 1/2 cup of turkey
- Kosher salt and Black Pepper to taste

Directions:
1. Heat the sesame oil in a minced pan. Attach the turkey and simmer till light brown, around seven minutes.
2. Add garlic, chili pepper, curry spice, and turmeric powder—cook 3 more minutes.
3. Add the milk and water, and feed. Season with black pepper and oil.
4. Cook at moderate heat for 45 minutes.

Nutrition:
Calories: 295
Fat: 2.9g
Carbohydrates: 0 g
Protein: 3.1g

50. Lettuce Wraps

Preparation Time: 10 minutes

Cooking Time: 10 minutes

Servings: 4

Ingredients:

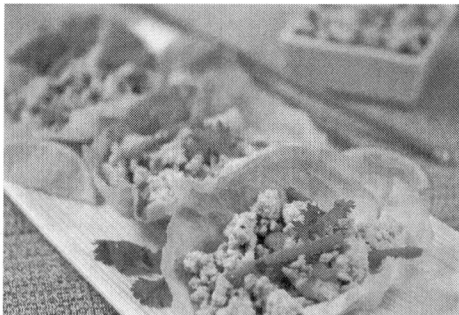

- 2 tablespoons soy sauce
- 1 teaspoon sesame oil
- 1 tablespoon olive oil
- 4 ounces water chestnuts, drained and diced
- 1 tablespoon fresh ginger, minced
- 1/2 cup hoisin sauce
- 1 1/2 tablespoons rice wine vinegar
- 1pound of ground chicken
- 1carrot, peeled and diced
- 2 teaspoons garlic, minced
- 2 teaspoons fresh ground ginger
- 2 small heads of butter lettuce
- 1/4 cup of sliced green onions, optional

Directions:

1. Put together the rice wine vinegar, soy sauce, hoisin sauce, and sesame oil in a tiny cup. Set it aside.
2. Clean the lettuce by rinsing it. Then, place the whole head of lettuce on a plate for quick picking, or separate the leaves and stack them.
3. Brown the ground chicken in olive oil over medium heat for around 6-7 minutes.
4. In a large mixing bowl, combine the diced carrots, garlic, ginger, and water chestnuts.
5. Before applying the hoisin sauce mixture, stir for around a minute. To add, mix thoroughly.
6. Prepare in a serving bowl and eat with the lettuce leaves or heads.

Nutrition:

Calories: 177   Fat: 11.2g Carbohydrates: 2.1g   Protein: 16.9g

Chapter 7.   Dinner Recipes

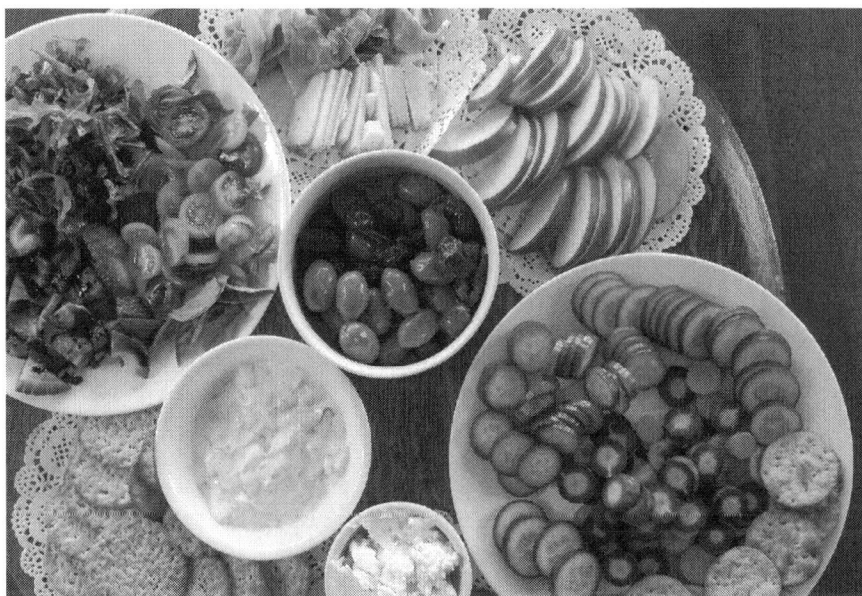

51. Zoodles with Keto Alfredo Sauce

Preparation Time: 10 minutes

Cooking Time: 10 minutes

Servings: 2

Ingredients:

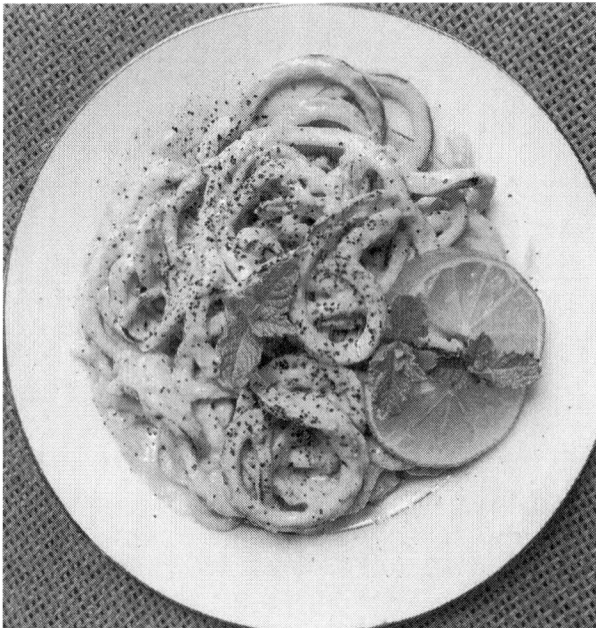

- 1 cup soaked, raw, unsalted cashews (reflected in nutrition) or 1 1/2 cups cooked cauliflower
- 1/2 cup homemade chicken bone broth
- 3 Tbsp. Bulletproof Grass-Fed Ghee or butter + extra for frying
- 2 Tbsp. Bulletproof Unflavored Collagen Powder
- 3/4 tsp. mustard powder
- 3/4 tsp. garlic powder
- 1/4-1/2 tsp. onion powder
- Salt, to taste
- 2 brown onions, diced
- 4-5 rashers of chemical-free bacon, diced
- 2 garlic cloves, crushed
- 2 medium-sized zucchini squashes

Directions:

1. Mix soaked (and strained) cashews or cooked cauliflower, bone broth, ghee (or butter), collagen powder, garlic, onion, and mustard powder in a mixer.
2. Blitz until smooth. It's about the taste. Then season with salt to taste.

3. In ghee, fry onions until golden brown. Cook bacon in the pan until it begins to crisp up.
4. Stir in the garlic, which has been crushed. Remove from heat until all ingredients are golden brown, and bacon is crispy.
5. In a medium saucepan, steam zoodles until they are cooked to your taste.
6. Meanwhile, warm the alfredo sauce in another small saucepan over medium heat.
7. Start plating until everything is packed. Divide the cooked zoodles into two bowls.
8. Serve with fried bacon and onions on top of the sauce. If required, top with fresh herbs and a pinch of salt and pepper.
9. Serve right away and enjoy!

Nutrition:

Calories: 209

Fat: 16g

Carbohydrates: 9g

Protein: 11g

52.   Kale Quinoa Salad

Preparation Time:
10 minutes
Cooking Time: 35
minutes
Servings: 2
Ingredients:

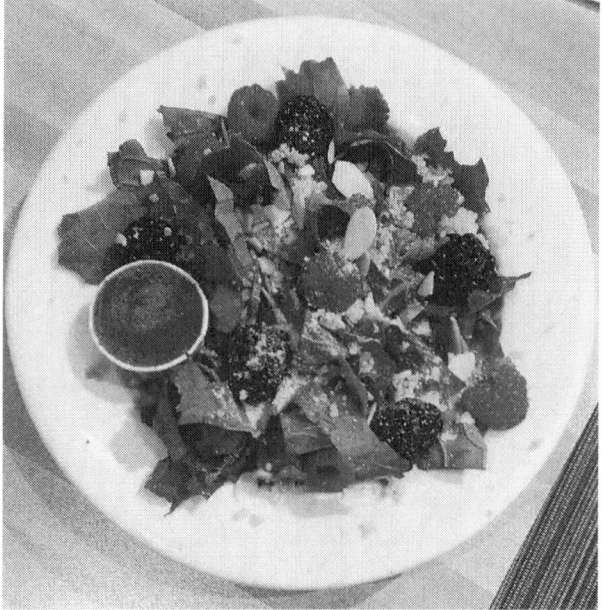

- 1 1/2 cups water
- 1/4 cup pine nuts (alternative: sunflower kernels)
- 1-piece small onion
- 1/2 cup tomato juice
- 1 cup quinoa rinsed
- 1 clove garlic
- 1/2 tsp red pepper flakes, crushed
- 6 cups fresh kale coarsely
- 1/4 cup raisins or dried cranberries
- 1 tbsp balsamic vinegar
- 1 tsp lemon juice
- 1 tsp grated lemon zest
- 1/4 tsp salt
- 1/8 tsp pepper
- 1 tbsp olive oil

Directions:

1. Minced the garlic, onion, and kale.
2. Wait for the water and tomato juice to boil in a big saucepan.
3. Reduce the heat and add the quinoa.
4. Put the cover and cook for 22 minutes, or until liquid has been consumed. Remove the quinoa from the heat and fluff with a fork.

5. Sauté onion in oil in a big skillet until tender.
6. Cook for an additional minute after adding the garlic and pepper flakes.
7. Cook for more minutes, or until the kale has wilted.
8. Combine pine nuts and raisins in a mixing bowl—Cook for more minutes or until the kale is tender.
9. Cook for a further 1-2 minutes after adding the vinegar, lemon juice, zest, salt, and pepper.
10. Get the pan from the heat and add the quinoa. Enable to cool before serving.

Nutrition:

Calories: 268

Fat: 8g

Carbohydrates: 46g

Protein: 7g

53.   Beef Stir Fry

Preparation Time: 5 minutes
Cooking Time: 15 minutes
Servings: 2
Ingredients:

- 1 tbsp olive oil
- 250 g beef sirloin, cut into strips
- 5 button mushrooms, sliced
- 1 cm fresh ginger, grated
- 1/2 tsp Chinese five-spice
- 1 garlic clove, peeled and crushed
- 200 g broccoli, cut into small florets
- 1 red pepper (capsicum), chopped
- 1 bunch Pak choi, chopped
- 1 1/2 tbsp tamari sauce
- sea salt
- black pepper

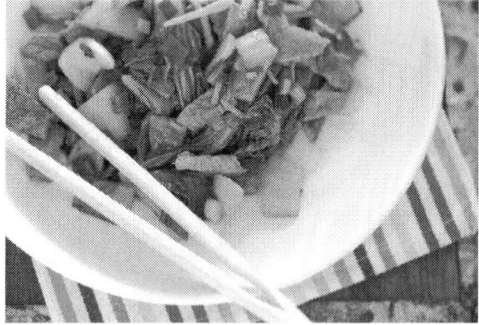

Directions:

1. In a big wok, heat half a tablespoon of olive oil over medium heat for around 2 minutes. Brown the beef in the wok, then cut it and set it aside.
2. Cook for about 4 minutes in the remaining olive oil with the mushrooms, ginger, five-spice, and garlic.
3. Cook for an extra 5 minutes after adding the broccoli, capsicum, and Pak choi.
4. Return the beef strips to the pan, stir in the soy sauce, and cook for another 2 minutes, or until heated through.
5. Divide the stir-fry in half and store it in an airtight tub in the refrigerator.
6. Place the remaining stir-fry half in a serving dish, season with salt and pepper, and serve.

Nutrition:

Calories: 370   Fat: 24g   Carbohydrates: 10g   Protein: 29g

54.   Turkey Sausage with Pepper and Onions

Preparation Time: 10 minutes
Cooking Time: 15 minutes
Servings: 2
Ingredients:
- 1-pound turkey rope sausage cut into thick half-moons
- 1/2 tablespoon olive oil
- 1 cup green pepper sliced
- 1 cup yellow pepper sliced
- 1 cup red onion sliced

Directions:
1. Put all the ingredients in a big skillet over medium-high heat.
2. Cook, often stirring, until the peppers and onions soften slightly.
3. Serve with quinoa or brown rice as a side dish. Have fun!

Nutrition:
Calories: 175
Fat: 11g
Carbohydrates: 7g
Protein: 13g

55.   Salmon and Bulgur Wheat Pilaf

Preparation Time: 20 minutes
Cooking Time: 30 minutes
Servings: 2
Ingredients:
- 1 lb. 1oz salmon, boned and skinned
- 8oz bulgur wheat
- 3oz frozen peas
- 7oz runner beans, chopped
- 2 tbsp chopped chives
- 2 tbsp chopped flat-leaf parsley
- salt and freshly ground black pepper
- 2 lemons halved
- 4 tbsp low-fat yogurt

Directions:
1. Prepare the oven to 350 F.
2. Cook the salmon for 15 minutes, wrapped in foil.
3. Meanwhile, in a medium-sized lidded jar, put the bulgur wheat. Then, 1cm/12 inches above the bulgur wheat, pour the boiling broth.
4. Place a cover and cook for 15 minutes over medium heat until the bulgur wheat is soft and has absorbed the liquid.
5. Cook the peas and beans until they're cooked to your taste in a pot of boiling water, then rinse.
6. Strip the salmon then toss it with the peas and beans in the bulgur wheat.
7. Combine the chives, parsley in a bowl, then salt and freshly ground black pepper to taste.
8. Serve with milk and lemon halves.

Nutrition:
Calories: 460
Fat: 14g
Carbohydrates: 49g
Protein: 32g

56.   Chicken with Red Kidney Beans

Preparation Time: 15 minutes

Cooking Time: 35 minutes

Servings: 2

Ingredients:

- 7oz easy-cook long-grain rice
- Cooking spray (low calorie)
- 1 chopped onion
- 1 chopped red pepper, cored, deseeded
- 1 garlic clove, cut in half
- 250 g skinless chicken thighs, cut into chunks
- 2 tsp. mild chili powder
- 400 g can of red kidney beans
- 400 g can of cherry tomatoes in natural juice
- 200 ml/7fl oz chicken stock
- Salt and freshly ground black pepper
- Fresh coriander leaves, roughly chopped
- Lime wedges

Directions:

1. Rinse and drain the red kidney beans.
2. Spray a large frying pan with a flameproof handle with oil and heat over medium heat.
3. Combine the onion, red pepper, garlic, and chicken in a large mixing bowl. Cook for 3 minutes and constantly stirring.
4. Preheat the grill to medium-high heat.
5. In a large skillet, combine the chili powder, flour, beans, tomatoes, and stock.
6. Season with salt and freshly ground black pepper to taste. Make it boil, then lower the heat and continue to cook for 15 minutes.
7. Heat the pan under the grill until golden brown.
8. Serve with lime wedges, divided among four plates, and garnished with coriander.

Nutrition:

Calories: 175   Fat: 1.7g

Carbohydrates: 15g   Protein: 25g

57. Quinoa Salad with Mint and Mango

Preparation Time: 20 minutes
Cooking Time: 30 minutes
Servings: 2
Ingredients:
- 4 oz quinoa, cooked according to packet Directions
- 1 tbsp chopped fresh mint
- 4 spring onions, including the green parts, chopped
- 2 tbsp chopped fresh coriander
- 1 mango, peeled, finely chopped
- 2 tbsp olive oil
- 1/2 lemon, juice only

Directions:
1. In a mixing cup, combine all of the ingredients and stir well.
2. Serve with surplus meats, such as grilled halloumi, chicken, or fish.

Nutrition:
Calories: 270
Fat: 4g
Carbohydrates: 54g
Protein: 10g

58.   Lemon and Pomegranate Couscous

Preparation   Time:
20 minutes

Cooking Time: 30 minutes

Servings: 2

Ingredients:

- 1 large or 2 small pomegranates
- 7oz couscous
- 250ml/9fl oz pints boiling chicken stock or water
- sea salt and freshly ground black pepper
- 2 lemons, juice only
- 6 tbsp olive oil
- 4 tbsp chopped, fresh mint or coriander

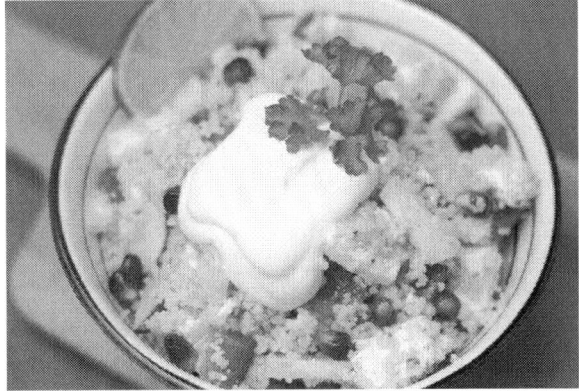

Directions:

1. Break the white membrane around the seeds by cutting the pomegranates in half and scooping out the seeds with a teaspoon.
2. In a dish, position the couscous. Pour the couscous with the boiling stock or water, then add the olive oil and lemon juice—season with freshly ground black pepper and sea salt.
3. Cover the couscous closely with plastic wrap and set aside for 5-10 minutes, or until the liquid has been absorbed.
4. Remove and use a fork to fluff the kernels. Allow for full cooling of the couscous.
5. Toss the couscous with the chopped herbs and pomegranate seeds.
6. To taste, add more olive oil, salt, pepper, and spices.

Nutrition:

Calories: 300

Fat: 17g

Carbohydrates: 31g

Protein: 5g

59. Tofu and Vegetable Skewers

Preparation Time: 1 hour
Cooking Time: 20 minutes
Servings: 4
Ingredients:

- 1/2 cup water (120 ml)
- 1/4 cup maple syrup (55 g)
- 3 tablespoons soy sauce
- 2 tablespoons BBQ sauce
- 1 tablespoon oil
- 1 tablespoon garlic powder
- 1 tablespoon sriracha
- 1 teaspoon black pepper
- 15 oz firm tofu (425 g) or extra firm tofu
- Pepper
- Onion
- Zucchini

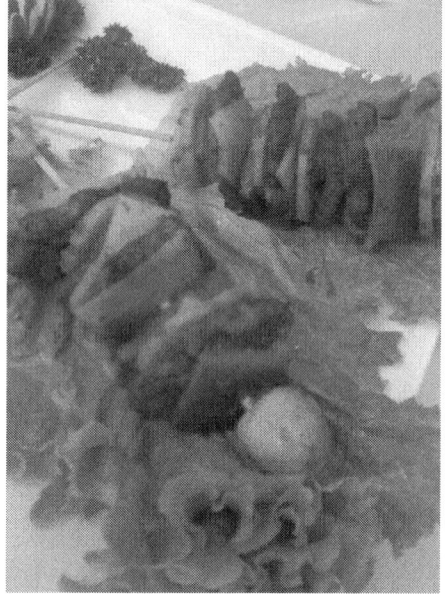

Directions:

1. To avoid fire, soak wooden skewers in a shallow dish of water.
2. Arrange the tofu on a plate lined with paper towels. Add another paper towel and a tray on top. 3 minutes in the microwave
3. Tofu can be cut into 9-12 cubes and put aside.
4. Stir together the water, maple syrup, soy sauce, barbecue sauce, oil, garlic powder, Sriracha, and pepper.
5. Put the tofu in the refrigerator for 1 hour after placing it in the marinade.
6. Let the tofu out of the marinade. Lower the heat, then cook for another 10 minutes before the marinade decreases and thickens.
7. Assemble the skewers, mixing tofu and vegetables.
8. Cook each skewer in a hot pan or grill for 4 minutes on each side.

Nutrition:
Calories: 277   Fat: 9g
Carbohydrates: 30g   Protein: 16g

60.   Black Olive and Tuna Salad

Preparation Time: 5 minutes
Cooking Time: 5 minutes
Servings: 2
Ingredients:

- 2 (5 to 6 oz.) Cans white tuna in water
- 1/4 cup chopped ripe pitted or Greek kalamata pitted olives
- 2 tablespoons olive oil
- 1 tablespoon balsamic vinegar
- 1 tablespoon fresh lemon juice
- 1/4 red onion, chopped
- 1 teaspoon capers (optional)
- Sea salt
- Ground black pepper, to taste

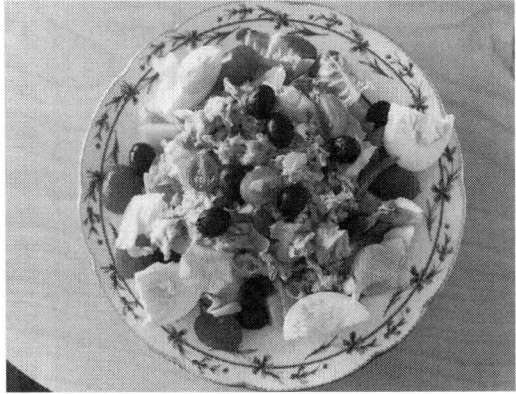

Directions:

1. Cut open the tuna cans with a can opener but keep the lids on. Holding the cans over a sink or a tub, press the tuna fish lid onto the tuna and tip the container to remove all of the oil.
2. Remove the lids from the tuna fish and place them in a big mixing bowl.
3. Toss the tuna fish with olives, oil, balsamic vinegar, lemon juice, red onion, capers (if using), salt, and some fresh black pepper.
4. Toss all together with a fork, breaking up any big bits of tuna as you go. Taste and adjust the amount of all of the ingredients to your liking.
5. Serve right away or keep refrigerated for up to 3 days in an airtight container.

Nutrition:
Calories: 217   Fat: 4g
Carbohydrates: 8g   Protein: 27g

61. Caprese Salad

Preparation Time: 10 minutes

Cooking Time: 15 minutes

Servings: 4 to 6

Ingredients:

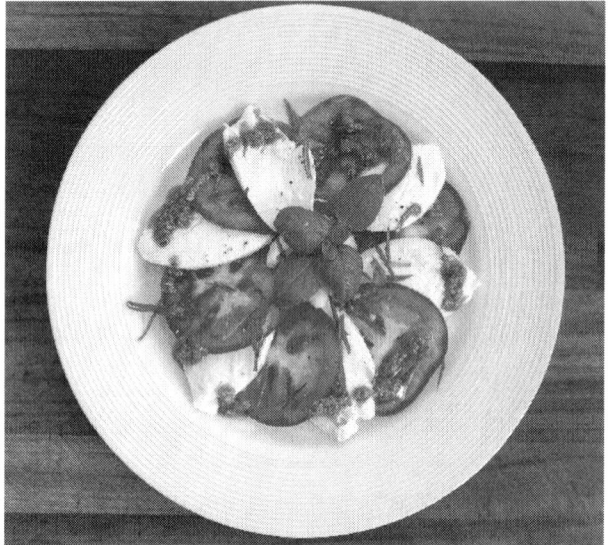

- 3 to 4 medium heirloom tomatoes, sliced
- 1 (8-ounce) ball fresh mozzarella, sliced
- 1/2 Fresh basil leaves
- 1/2 Extra-virgin olive oil for drizzling
- Sea salt and ground black pepper

Optional additions/variations:

- Drizzle of balsamic vinegar or reduced balsamic
- 1/2 Dollops of pesto
- 1/2 Mint leaves
- 2 small Sliced peaches
- 1 small Avocado slice
- 1/2 cup Strawberries

Directions:

1. Spread tomatoes, mozzarella, and basil leaves on a platter.
2. Put some olive oil and sprinkle with sea salt and ground black pepper.
3. If desired, add ingredients from the variations list.

Nutrition:

Calories: 150   Fat: 10g

Carbohydrates: 2g   Protein: 8g

62.   Beans and Cheese on Toast

Preparation Time: 5 minutes
Cooking Time: 15 minutes
Servings: 4
Ingredients:
- 4 slices Co-op farmhouse loaf
- 1 x 420g Co-op baked beans
- 60g Co-op mature Cheddar cheese, grated

Directions:
1. Cook the beans according to the package instructions.
2. Serve with lots of grated cheese on top of hot buttered toast.
3. Until eating, make sure your meal is thoroughly cooked and piping hot.

Nutrition:
Calories: 440
Fat: 11g
Carbohydrates: 63g
Protein: 19g

63.   Fried Whole Tilapia

Preparation time: 10 minutes.
Cooking time: 25 minutes.
Servings: 2
Ingredients:

- 10 ounces tilapia
- 2 tablespoons oil
- 4 large onion, chopped
- 2 garlic cloves, minced
- 2 tablespoons red chili powder
- 1 teaspoon turmeric powder
- 1 teaspoon cumin powder
- 1 teaspoon coriander powder
- Salt to taste
- Black pepper to taste
- 2 tablespoons soy sauce
- 2 tablespoons fish sauce

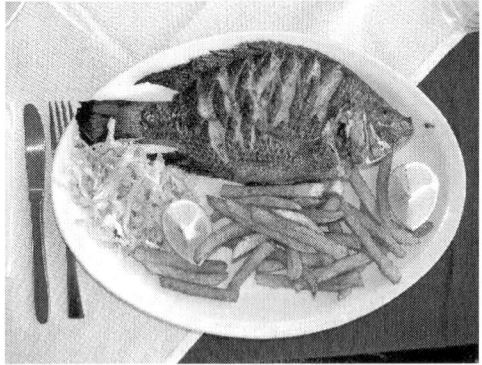

Directions:

1. Take the tilapia fish and clean it well without taking off the skin. You need to fry it whole, so you have to be careful about cleaning the gut inside.
2. Cut few slits on the skin so the seasoning gets inside well.
3. Marinate the fish with fish sauce, soy sauce, red chili powder, garlic, cumin powder, turmeric powder, coriander powder, salt, and pepper.
4. Coat half of the onions in the same mixture too.
5. Let them marinate for 1 hour.
6. In a skillet, heat the oil. Fry the fish for 8 minutes on each side.
7. Transfer the fish to a serving plate.
8. Fry the marinated onions until they become crispy.
9. Add the remaining raw onions on top and serve hot.

Nutrition:

Calories: 368   Fat: 30.1g   Carbohydrates: 9.2g   Protein: 16.6g

64.   Garlic Chicken Livers

Preparation time: 10 minutes
Cooking time: 30 minutes
Servings: 2
Ingredients:
- 1/2-pound chicken liver
- 6 garlic cloves, minced
- 1/2 teaspoon salt
- 1 tablespoon ginger garlic paste
- 1 cup diced onion
- 1 tablespoon red chili powder
- 1 teaspoon cumin
- 1 teaspoon coriander powder
- Black pepper to taste
- 1 cardamom
- 2 tomatoes
- 1 cinnamon stick
- 1 bay leaf
- 4 tablespoons olive oil
- 2 tablespoons lemon juice

Directions:
1. Get a large pan, warm your oil over high heat.
2. Add the garlic and fry them golden brown.
3. Add onion and fry until they become caramelized.
4. Change the heat to medium, then add the bay leaf, cinnamon stick, cardamom, and toss for 30 seconds.
5. Add the ginger-garlic paste and 1 tablespoon of water. Adding water prevents burning.
6. Add the coriander powder, black pepper, salt, cumin, and red chili powder.
7. Cover and cook for 3 minutes on low heat.
8. Add the livers and 2 tablespoons of lemon juice cook on medium heat for 15 minutes.
9. Add the tomatoes and cook for another 5 minutes.
10. Check the seasoning. Add more salt if needed.

11. Serve hot with a tortilla.

Nutrition:

Calories: 174

Fat: 9g

Protein: 18g

Carbohydrates: 2.4g

65. Healthy Chickpea Burger

Preparation time: 15 minutes

Cooking time: 10 minutes

Servings: 2

Ingredients:

- 1 cup chickpeas, boiled
- 1 tablespoon tomato puree
- 1 teaspoon soy sauce
- A pinch of paprika
- A pinch of white pepper
- 1 onion, diced
- Salt to taste
- 2 lettuce leaves
- 1/2 cup bell pepper, sliced
- 1 teaspoon olive oil
- 1 avocado, sliced
- 2 burger buns to serve

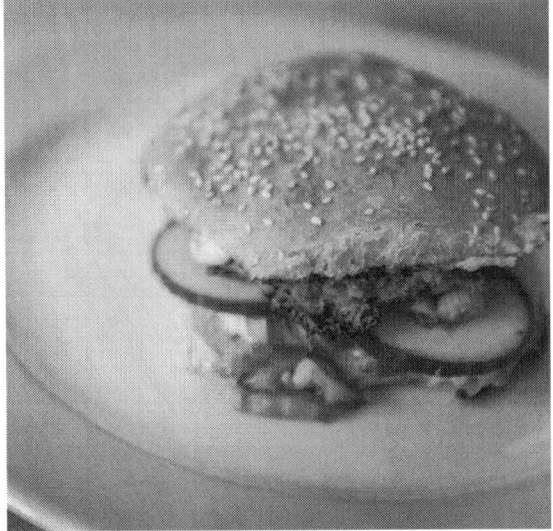

Directions:

1. Mash the chickpeas and combine them with bell pepper, salt, pepper, paprika, soy sauce, and tomato puree.
2. Use your hands to make patties.
3. Fry the patties golden brown with oil.
4. Assemble the burgers with lettuce, onion, and avocado and enjoy.

Nutrition:

Calories: 254

Fat: 12g

Protein: 9g

Carbohydrates: 7.8g

66. Southwest Chicken Salad

Preparation time: 15 minutes

Cooking time: 15 minutes

Servings: 8

Ingredients:

- 1/4 cup extra-virgin olive oil
- 1/4 cup red onion, finely chopped
- 1 cup corn, drained
- 1 can low-sodium black beans, rinsed and drained
- 1 jalapeno, seeded and minced
- 1 teaspoon chili powder
- 1 teaspoon cumin
- 1 teaspoon garlic powder
- 1 teaspoon onion powder
- 2 bell peppers, diced
- 2 large limes, juiced
- 2 pounds chicken thighs, cooked and diced
- 2 tablespoons cilantro, finely chopped
- 3 cups quinoa, cooked
- Sea salt and black pepper to taste

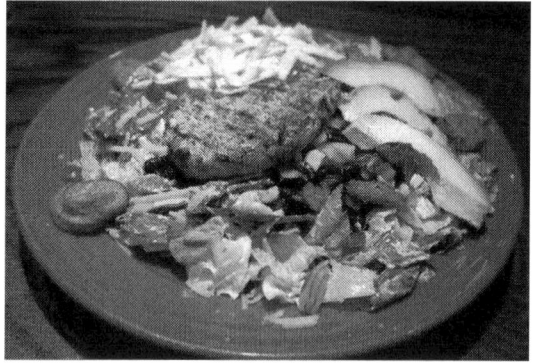

Directions:

1. In a mixing bowl, place chili powder, lime juice, onion powder, garlic powder, cumin, and cilantro. Mix thoroughly and put aside.
2. Get another bowl, put all the other ingredients, and toss until thoroughly combined.
3. Drizzle seasoning mixture over the salad and toss to coat thoroughly.
4. Place a cover and let it cool for 30 minutes before serving.

Nutrition:

Calories: 217   Carbohydrates: 30g   Fat: 9g   Protein: 7g

67.   Calamari Rings

Preparation   time:
5 minutes

Cooking time: 2
minutes

Servings: 4

Ingredients:

- 4 calamari squid tubes
- 1 tablespoon ghee
- 2 tablespoons almond flour
- Zest and juice of 1 lemon
- Salt and pepper to taste

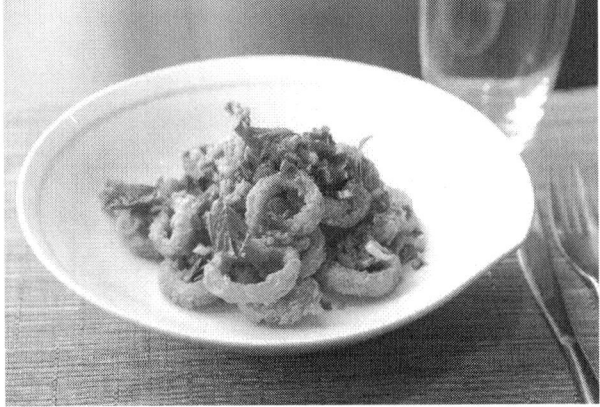

Directions:

1. Mix the almond flour, lemon zest, salt, and pepper.
2. Slice the squid tubes into 1/2-inch slices.
3. Roll the calamari rings in the almond mix.
4. Heat ghee in a frying pan and fry rings on low heat for 1 minute on each side until cooked and golden.
5. Drizzle with lemon juice.

Nutrition:

Carbohydrates: 5.9g

Fat: 8.2g

Protein: 16.3g

Calories: 159

68.   Zucchini Avocado Carpaccio

Preparation time: 10 minutes
Cooking time: 5 minutes
Servings: 2
Ingredients:

- 3 cups thinly sliced zucchini
- 1 thinly sliced ripe avocado
- 1 tablespoon freshly squeezed lemon juice
- 1 tablespoon extra-virgin olive oil
- 1/4 tablespoon finely grated lemon zest
- 1/2 teaspoon freshly ground black pepper
- 1-ounce sliced and chopped almonds
- Sea salt to taste

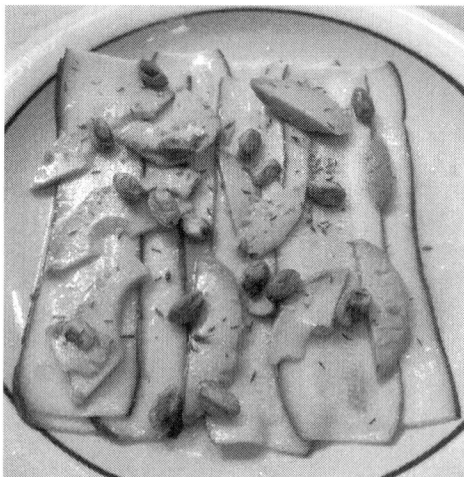

Directions:

1. Mix the lemon juice with the lemon zest in a bowl. Add in the olive oil along with black pepper and sea salt.
2. Thinly slice the zucchini and avocado on a plate.
3. Set the avocado and zucchini and on a plate in an overlapping manner.
4. Now, drizzle the lemon juice mixture over the salad.
5. Top the salad with finely chopped almonds.

Nutrition:

Calories: 81

Carbohydrates: 5g

Fat: 6g

Protein: 3g

69. Slow Cooker Eggplant Bacon Wraps

Preparation time: 15 minutes

Cooking time: 5 hours

Servings: 6

Ingredients:
- 10 ounces eggplant, sliced into rounds
- 5 ounces Halloumi cheese
- 1 teaspoon minced garlic
- 3 ounces bacon, chopped
- 1/2 teaspoon ground black pepper
- 1 teaspoon salt
- 1 teaspoon paprika
- 1 tomato

Directions:
1. Rub the eggplant slices with the ground black pepper, salt, and paprika.
2. Slice Halloumi cheese and tomato.
3. Combine the chopped bacon and minced garlic together.
4. Place the sliced eggplants in the slow cooker—Cook the eggplant on high for 1 hour.
5. Chill the eggplant. Place the sliced tomato and cheese on the eggplant slices.
6. Add the chopped bacon mixture and roll up tightly.
7. Secure the eggplants with the toothpicks and return the eggplant wraps into the slow cooker—Cook the dish for 4 hours more on a high mode.
8. When the dish is done, serve it immediately. Enjoy!

Nutrition:

Calories: 131

Fat: 9.4g

Carbohydrates: 7.25g

Protein: 6g

70. Slow Cooker Stuffed Eggplants

Preparation time: 20 minutes
Cooking time: 8 hours
Servings: 4
Ingredients:

- 4 medium eggplants
- 1 cup rice, half-cooked
- 1/2 cup chicken stock
- 1 teaspoon salt
- 1 teaspoon paprika
- 1/2 cup fresh cilantro
- 3 tablespoons tomato sauce
- 1 teaspoon olive oil

Directions:

1. Wash the eggplants carefully and remove the flesh from them.
2. Then combine the rice with salt, paprika, and tomato sauce.
3. Chop the fresh cilantro and add it to the rice mixture.
4. Then, fill the prepared eggplants with the rice mixture.
5. Pour the chicken stock and olive oil into the slow cooker.
6. Add the stuffed eggplants and close the slow cooker lid. Cook the dish on low for 8 hours.
7. When the eggplants are done, chill them a little and serve immediately. Enjoy!

Nutrition:
Calories: 277
Fat: 9.1g
Carbohydrates: 51.92g
Protein: 11g

71. Cobb Salad

Preparation time: 12 minutes

Cooking time: 8 minutes

Servings: 2

Ingredients:

- 1 hard-boiled egg, sliced
- 1 avocado, halved and sliced
- 1/2 cup sliced cherry tomatoes (optional)
- 1 cup cubed or shredded chicken breast
- 4 slices of cooked bacon, chopped
- 1/4 cup broken blue cheese
- 2 tablespoons sliced green onions (optional)
- 1 head of lettuce, leaves separated
- Olive oil to taste
- Lemon juice to taste

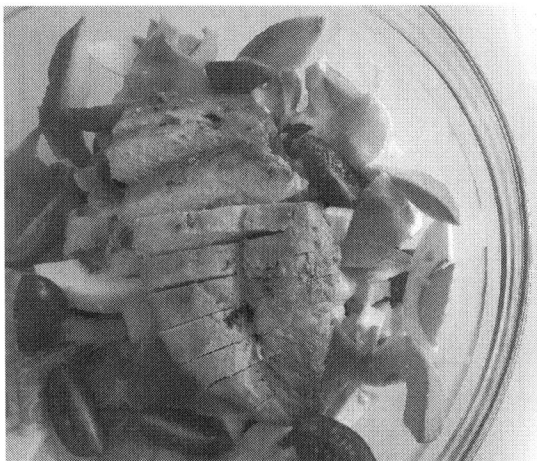

Directions:

1. In a big deep dish, toss with the egg, avocado, tomatoes if using chicken, bacon, blue cheese, and green onions.
2. Place on the lettuce.
3. Sprinkle in olive oil and lemon juice to taste or use any salad dressing you like.

Nutrition:

Calories: 290

Fat: 15g

Carbohydrates: 5g

Protein: 16g

72.   Tuna Salad

Preparation time: 15 minutes

Cooking time: 5 minutes

Servings: 4

Ingredients:

- 1/4 cup mayonnaise
- 1/4 cup red onion, finely diced
- 3/4 cup plain yogurt
- 1 clove garlic, minced
- 1 large , diced
- 1 tablespoon lemon juice
- 2 small dill pickles, diced
- 24 ounces tuna packed in water, drained
- Sea salt and pepper to taste

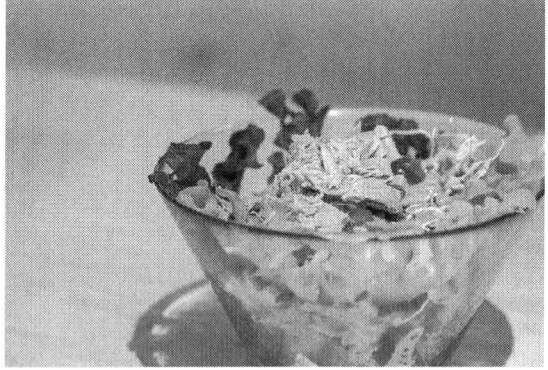

Directions:

1. Prepare a mixing bowl, combine all the ingredients, and stir to combine thoroughly.
2. Cover and chill for at least 15 minutes before serving.
3. Serve chilled!

Nutrition:

Calories: 152

Carbohydrates: 2g

Fat: 8g

Protein: 18g

73. Black Bean and Quinoa Salad

Preparation time: 15 minutes

Cooking time: 15 minutes

Servings: 4

Ingredients:

- 3 cups quinoa
- 14 ounces low-sodium black beans
- 1 large tomato, diced
- 2 tablespoons cilantro, finely chopped
- 1/4 cup red onion, finely diced
- 1 jalapeno, seeded and minced
- 1 clove garlic, minced
- 2 large limes, juiced
- 1/4 cup extra-virgin olive oil
- 1 teaspoon cumin
- 1 teaspoon chili powder
- 1 teaspoon onion powder
- Sea salt and pepper to taste

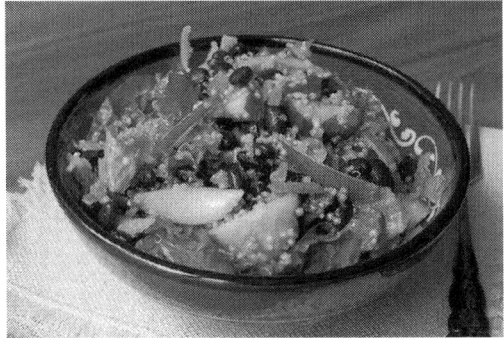

Directions:

1. Rinse and drain the black beans.
2. Prepare the quinoa following the package instructions and let it cool.
3. Get a small bowl, put in the olive oil, lime juice, cumin, cilantro, salt, pepper, chili powder, and onion powder. Mix thoroughly.
4. Get a large mixing bowl, put together the remaining ingredients and stir to combine thoroughly.
5. Drizzle dressing over the mixture and stir once more to combine.
6. Put a cover before chilling the salad for 15 minutes before serving. Serve chilled!

Nutrition:

Calories: 261   Carbohydrates: 38g

Fat: 8g   Protein: 10g

74. Thai-Inspired Chicken Salad

Preparation time: 10 minutes
Cooking time: 15 minutes
Servings: 8
Ingredients:

- 1/4 cup cilantro, finely chopped
- 1/4 cup green onion, chopped
- 1/2 peanuts, roasted and unsalted
- 1/2 teaspoon red pepper flakes
- 1 cup plain yogurt
- 1 medium bell pepper, diced
- 2 cups red cabbage, chopped
- 2 chicken breasts, cooked and shredded
- 2 tablespoons maple syrup
- 3 tablespoons rice wine vinegar
- Sea salt and pepper to taste

Directions:

1. In a medium bowl, place all the ingredients and stir to combine thoroughly.
2. Cover and chill for at least 15 minutes before serving.
3. Serve chilled!

Nutrition:
Calories: 152
Carbohydrates: 2g
Fat: 8g
Protein: 18g

75. Slow Cooker Chicken Open Sandwich

Preparation time: 15 minutes
Cooking time: 8 hours
Servings: 4
Ingredients:
- 7 ounces chicken fillet
- 1 teaspoon cayenne pepper
- 5 ounces mashed potato, cooked
- 6 tablespoons chicken gravy
- 4 slices French bread, toasted
- 2 teaspoons mayo
- 1 cup water

Directions:
1. Put the chicken fillet in the slow cooker and sprinkle it with cayenne pepper.
2. Add water and chicken gravy. Close the slow cooker cover and let it cook the chicken for 8 hours on low.
3. Then combine the mashed potato with the mayo sauce. Spread toasted French bread with the mashed potato mixture.
4. Once cooked, cut it into strips and combine it with the remaining gravy from the slow cooker.
5. Place the chicken strips over the mashed potato.
6. Enjoy the open sandwich warm!

Nutrition:
Calories: 285
Fat: 7g
Carbohydrates: 27g
Protein: 27g

Chapter 8. Vegetarian Recipes and Others

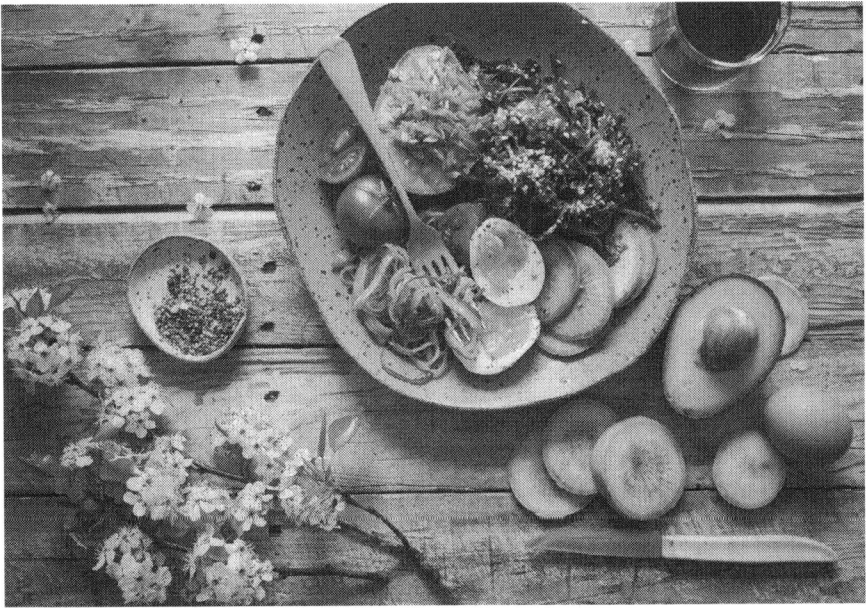

76. Roasted Brussels Sprouts with Pecans and Gorgonzola

Preparation time: 10 minutes
Cooking time: 35 minutes
Servings: 4
Ingredients:

- 1-pound Brussels sprouts, fresh
- 1/4 cup pecans, chopped
- 1 tablespoon olive oil
- Extra olive oil to grease the baking tray
- Pepper and salt for tasting
- 1/4 cup Gorgonzola cheese

(If you prefer not to use the Gorgonzola cheese, you can toss the Brussels sprouts when hot, with 2 tablespoons of butter instead)

Directions:

1. Warm the oven to 350 F.
2. Rub a large pan with a bit of olive oil. You can use a pastry brush or paper towel.
3. Cut off the ends of the Brussels sprouts if you need to, and then cut them lengthwise into halves.
4. Chop up all the pecans using a knife and then measure them for the amount.
5. Put your Brussels sprouts as well as the sliced pecans inside a bowl and cover them all with some olive oil, pepper, and salt.
6. Arrange all of your pecans and Brussels sprouts onto your roasting pan in a single layer.
7. Roast this for 30 to 35 minutes, or when they become tender and can be pierced with a fork easily. Stir during cooking if you wish to get a more even browning.
8. Once cooked, toss them with the Gorgonzola cheese (or butter) before you serve them. Serve them hot.

Nutrition:
Calories: 149   Fat: 11g
Carbohydrates: 10g   Protein: 5g

77. Artichoke Petals Bites

Preparation time: 10 minutes
Cooking time: 10 minutes
Servings: 8
Ingredients:
- 8 ounces artichoke petals, boiled, drained, without salt
- 1/2 cup almond flour
- 4 ounces Parmesan, grated
- 2 tablespoons almond butter, melted

Directions:
1. In the mixing bowl, mix up together almond flour and grated parmesan.
2. Prepare the oven to 355 F.
3. Dip the artichoke petals in the almond butter and then coat in the almond flour mixture.
4. Place them on the tray.
5. Move the tray to the preheated oven and cook the petals for 10 minutes.
6. Chill the cooked petal bites a little before serving.

Nutrition:
Calories: 93
Protein: 6.54g
Fat: 3.72g
Carbohydrates: 9.08g

78. Eggplant Fries

Preparation time: 10 minutes

Cooking time: 15 minutes

Servings: 8

Ingredients:

- 2 eggs
- 2 cups almond flour
- 2 tablespoons coconut oil, spray
- 2 eggplant, peeled and cut thinly
- Salt and pepper to taste

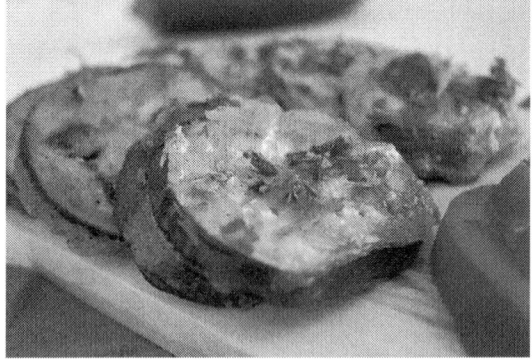

Directions:

1. Prepare the oven to 400 F.
2. Take a bowl and mix with salt and black pepper in it.
3. Take another bowl and beat eggs until frothy.
4. Dip the eggplant pieces into eggs.
5. Then coat them with a flour mixture.
6. Add another layer of flour and egg.
7. Then, take a baking sheet and grease with coconut oil on top.
8. Bake for about 15 minutes. Serve and enjoy.

Nutrition:

Calories: 212

Fat: 15.8g

Carbohydrates: 12.1g

Protein: 8.6g

79.   Roasted Broccoli

Preparation time: 5
minutes
Cooking time: 20
minutes
Servings: 4
Ingredients:

- 4 cups broccoli
  florets
- 1 tablespoon
  olive oil
- Salt and pepper to taste

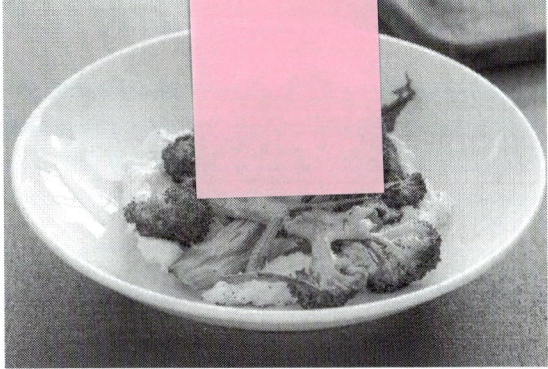

Directions:

1. Preheat your oven to 400 F.
2. Add broccoli in a zip bag alongside oil and shake until coated.
3. Add seasoning and shake again.
4. Spread the broccoli out on the baking sheet and bake for 20 minutes.
5. Let it cool and serve.

Nutrition:
Calories: 62
Fat: 4g
Carbohydrates: 4g
Protein: 4g

80. Squash Bites

Preparation time: 10 minutes
Cooking time: 40 minutes
Servings: 4
Ingredients:

- 10 ounces of turkey meat, cooked, sliced
- 2 pounds butternut squash, cubed
- 1 teaspoon chili powder
- 1 teaspoon garlic powder
- 1 teaspoon sweet paprika
- Black pepper to taste

Directions:

1. In a bowl, mix butternut squash cubes with chili powder, black pepper, garlic powder, paprika, and toss to coat.
2. Wrap squash pieces in turkey slices, place them all on a lined baking sheet.
3. Set and bake in the oven at 350 F for 20 minutes, flip and bake for 20 minutes more.
4. Arrange squash bites on a platter and serve. Enjoy!

Nutrition:
Calories: 223
Fat: 3.8g
Carbohydrates: 26.5g
Protein: 23g

81.   Zucchini Chips

Preparation time: 10 minutes
Cooking time: 12 minutes
Servings: 4
Ingredients:

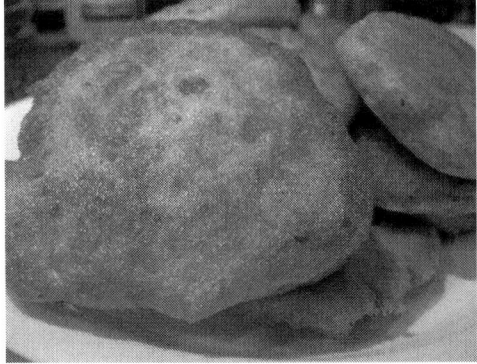

- 1 zucchini, thinly sliced
- A pinch of sea salt
- Black pepper to taste
- 1 teaspoon thyme, dried
- 1 egg
- 1 teaspoon garlic powder
- 1 cup almond flour

Directions:

1. In a mixing bowl, whisk together the egg and a pinch of salt.
2. In a separate bowl, combine the flour, thyme, black pepper, and garlic powder.
3. Dredge zucchini slices in flour and then in the egg mixture.
4. Place the chips on a prepared baking sheet and bake for 6 minutes on each side at 450 degrees F.
5. Serve the zucchini chips as a snack. Enjoy!

Nutrition:

Calories: 106
Fat: 8.2g
Carbohydrates: 5.2g
Protein: 5.1g

82.   Italian-Style Asparagus with Cheese

Preparation time: 10 minutes
Cooking time: 10 minutes
Servings: 2
Ingredients:
- 1/2-pound asparagus spears, trimmed, cut into bite-sized pieces
- 1 teaspoon Italian spice blend
- 1/2 tablespoon lemon juice
- 1 tablespoon extra-virgin olive oil
- 4 tablespoons Romano cheese, freshly grated

Directions:
1. Prepare a saucepan with lightly salted water and wait for a boil. Turn the heat to medium-low.
2. Add the asparagus spears and cook for approximately 3 minutes.
3. Drain and transfer to a serving bowl.
4. Add the Italian spice blend, lemon juice, and extra-virgin olive oil; toss until well coated.
5. Top with the Romano cheese and serve immediately. Serve.

Nutrition:
Calories: 193
Fat: 14.1g
Carbohydrates: 5.6g
Protein: 11.5g

83. Cheddar Cauliflower Bites

Preparation time: 10 minutes
Cooking time: 25 minutes
Servings: 8
Ingredients:
- 1-pound cauliflower florets
- 1 teaspoon sweet paprika
- A pinch of salt and black pepper
- 2 eggs, whisked
- 1 cup coconut flour
- Cooking spray for spraying
- 1 cup Cheddar cheese, grated

Directions:
1. In a bowl put together the flour with salt, pepper, cheese, and paprika and stir.
2. Put the eggs in a separate bowl.
3. Dredge the cauliflower florets in the eggs and then in the cheese mix.
4. Prepare a baking sheet with parchment paper. Arrange florets, then bake at 360 F for 25 minutes.
5. Serve as a snack.

Nutrition:
Calories: 163
Fat: 12g
Carbohydrates: 2g
Protein: 7g

84.   Herbed Coconut Flour Bread

Preparation time: 10 minutes

Cooking time: 3 minutes

Servings: 2

Ingredients:

- 4 tablespoons coconut flour
- 1/2 teaspoon baking powder
- 1/2 teaspoon dried thyme
- 2 tablespoons whipping cream
- 2 eggs

Seasoning:

- 1/2 teaspoon oregano
- 2 tablespoons avocado oil

Directions:

1. Take a medium bowl, place all the ingredients in it, and then whisk until incorporated and smooth batter comes together.
2. Distribute the mixture evenly between two mugs and then microwave for a minute and 30 seconds until cooked.
3. When done, take out bread from the mugs, cut it into slices, and then serve.

Nutrition:

Calories: 309

Fats: 26.1g

Protein: 9.3g

Carbohydrates: 4.3g

85. Minty Zucchinis

Preparation time: 10 minutes
Cooking time: 15 minutes
Servings: 4
Ingredients:
- 1-pound zucchinis, sliced
- 1 tablespoon olive oil
- 2 garlic cloves, minced
- 1 tablespoon mint, chopped
- Pinch of salt and black pepper
- 1/4 cup veggie stock

Directions:
1. Heat a pan with the oil over medium-high heat and add garlic and sauté for 2 minutes.
2. Add the zucchinis and the other ingredients, toss, cook everything for 10 minutes more.
3. Serve as a side dish.

Nutrition:
Calories: 70
Fat: 1g
Carbohydrates: 0.4g
Protein: 6g

86. Almond Flour Muffins

Preparation time: 15 minutes

Cooking time: 30 minutes

Servings: 8

Ingredients:

- 1/3 cup of pumpkin puree
- 3 eggs
- 2 tablespoons agave nectar
- 2 tablespoons coconut oil
- 1 teaspoon vanilla extract
- 1 teaspoon white vinegar
- 1 cup chopped fruits
- 1 teaspoon baking soda
- 1/2 teaspoon salt
- 2 tablespoons of Almond flour

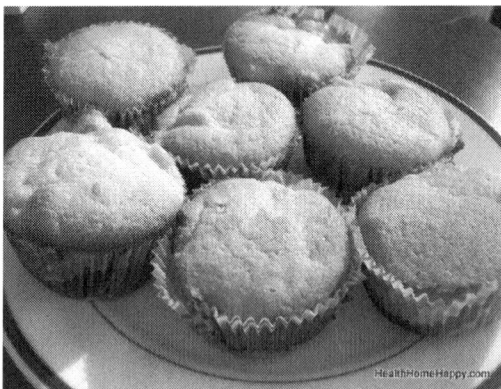

Directions:

1. Preheat the oven to 350 F.
2. Prepare a muffin tin with paper liners.
3. In the first mixing bowl, whisk the almond flour, salt, and baking soda.
4. In the second mixing bowl, whisk the pumpkin puree, eggs, coconut oil, agave nectar, vanilla extract, and vinegar.
5. Now add this puree mix of the second bowl to the first bowl and blend everything well.
6. Add the chopped fruits to the blend.
7. Pour the mixture into the muffin cups in your pan.
8. Bake for 15–20 minutes. Ensure that the contents have been set in the center, and a golden-brown lining has started to appear at the edges.
9. Place muffins to a cooling rack and let them cool completely.

Nutrition:

Calories: 173   Carbohydrates: 4g   Fat: 16g   Protein: 4g

87. Parmesan Crisps

Preparation time: 5 minutes

Cooking time: 25 minutes

Servings: 8

Ingredients:

- 1 teaspoon butter
- 8 ounces parmesan cheese, full fat, and shredded

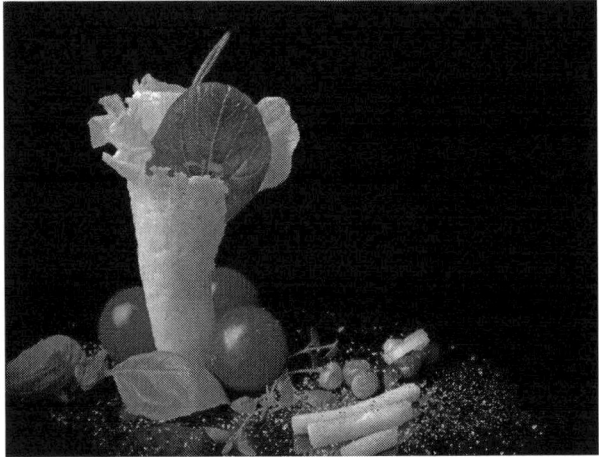

Directions:

1. Preheat the oven to 400 F.
2. Place a parchment paper on a baking sheet and grease with butter.
3. Spoon parmesan into 8 mounds, spreading them apart evenly. Flatten them.
4. Bake for 5 minutes until browned.
5. Let them cool. Serve and enjoy.

Nutrition:

Calories: 133

Fat: 11g

Carbohydrates: 1g

Protein: 11g

88. Broccoli Salad

Preparation Time:
20 minutes
Cooking Time: 5
minutes
Servings: 6
Ingredients:

- 1/2 cup of pecans, chopped
- 1 and a half tablespoons. onion powder
- 1 pound of broccoli
- 1/2 pound of mushrooms
- 1 small pepper, cut into strips
- 1 tablespoon. apple cider vinegar
- 2 tbsp of toasted sesame seeds
- 2 tbsp of extra virgin olive oil
- Sea salt and pepper, just enough

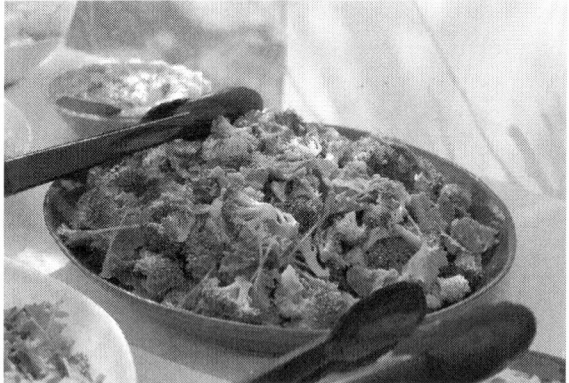

Directions:

1. Heat the pan well with oil and sauté the broccoli and pepperoni.
2. Add the mushrooms and cook until the broccoli is tender.
3. Leave the mixture to rest for 15 min.
4. In a medium bowl, mix all ingredients thoroughly.
5. Serve immediately!

Nutrition:
Calories 250
Carbohydrates 20g
Fats 16g
Protein12g

89.   Cabbage Casserole

Preparation Time: 10 minutes
Cooking Time: 55 minutes
Servings: 6
Ingredients:

- 1/2 head cabbage
- 2 scallions, chopped
- 2 grated carrots
- 4 tablespoons unsalted butter
- 2 ounces cream cheese, softened
- 1/4 cup Parmesan cheese, grated
- 1/4 cup fresh cream
- 1/2 teaspoon Dijon mustard
- 2 tablespoons fresh parsley, chopped
- Salt and ground black pepper, as required

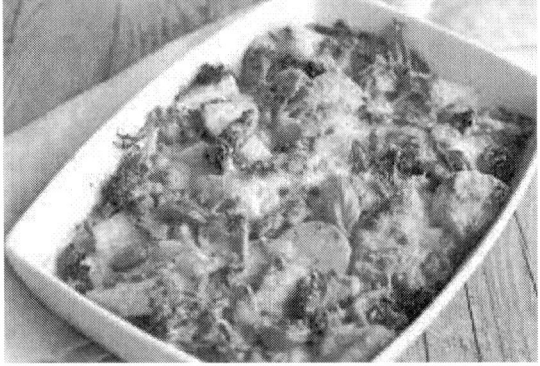

Directions:

1. Prepare the oven to 350 F.
2. Cut the cabbage head into half lengthwise. Then cut into 4 equal-sized wedges.
3. In a deep pot of boiling water, add cabbage wedges and cook, covered for about 5 minutes.
4. Drain well and arrange cabbage wedges into a small baking dish.
5. In a small pan, melt butter and sauté onions for about 5 minutes.
6. Add the remaining ingredients and stir to combine.
7. Remove from the heat and immediately place the cheese mixture over cabbage wedges evenly.
8. Bake for about 20 mins.
9. Get the casserole from the oven and let it cool for about 5 minutes before serving.
10. Cut into 3 equal-sized portions and serve.

Nutrition:

Calories 273   Fat 8g   Carbohydrates 8g   Protein 9g

90.   Ginger Orange Stir-fry with Tofu

<u>Preparation Time</u>: 25 minutes
<u>Cooking Time</u>: 30 minutes
<u>Servings</u>: 4
<u>Ingredients</u>:

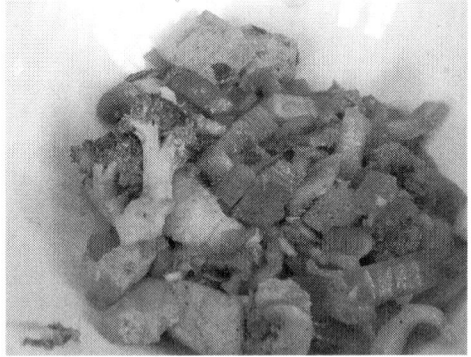

- 1 bunch of broccolis, cut into florets
- 1 block of organic extra-firm tofu, cut into 1/2 – inch cubes
- 1 tablespoon fresh ginger, grated
- 2 cloves of garlic
- 1/4 cup of coconut sugar
- 2 tablespoons Tamari
- 1 tablespoon of rice wine vinegar
- 1/2 cup of water
- 1 tablespoon arrowroot starch
- 1 cup of frozen edamame
- 2 tablespoons Unrefined coconut oil
- 1/2 cup of raw cashews
- 2 green onions, chopped
- 1 tablespoon of sesame seeds
- 1 cup of fresh orange juice
- 4 servings of cooked brown rice

<u>Directions</u>:

1. Place fruit juice in a very tiny pan over medium heat. Add the garlic, ginger, tamari, coconut sugar, and vinegar.
2. Mix well and maintain heat until it simmers. Reduce heat to low to take care of a delicate simmer. Continue to cook for another 10 minutes.
3. Set a saucepan in medium-high heat and heat coconut oil. Sauté tofu for 5 minutes until slightly browned.
4. Add the edamame and broccoli. Continue to sauté another 5 minutes or until the broccoli is tender.

5. Dissolve arrowroot starch in water. Add it to the ginger-orange sauce and adjust heat to medium while whisking continuously.

6. Cook another minute or until the consistency thickens. Remove the pan from the heat.

7. Pour the sauce over the tofu and vegetables. Add the cashews and mix well. Remove pan from heat.

8. To serve, pour over brown rice. Top with green onions and sesame seeds.

Nutrition:

Calories 160

Fat 8g

Carbohydrates 12g

Protein 12g

91.   Cauliflower Mashed Potatoes

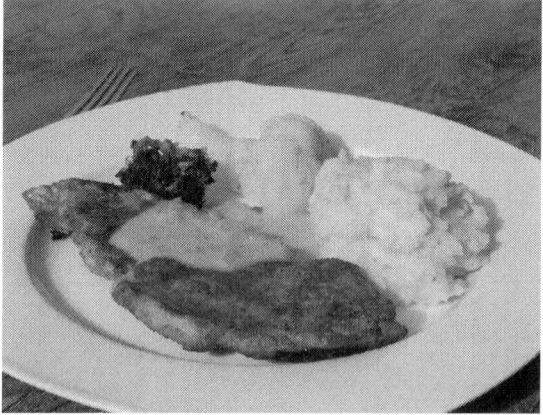

Preparation Time: 10 minutes

Cooking Time: 22 minutes

Servings: 3

Ingredients:
- 1 cup of chopped cauliflower
- 2 tablespoons of heavy cream
- 2 tablespoons of melted butter
- 1 tablespoon of mayonnaise
- 1/2 teaspoon of salt

Directions:
1. Set your oven to 375 F.
2. While your oven is heating up, place your 1 cup of chopped cauliflower into a heat resistant bowl followed by your 2 tablespoons of water. Drizzle on the cauliflower just to make sure that it maintains moisture.
3. Cook in the microwave for about 3 minutes.
4. Now, take out of the microwave, deposit cauliflower into a blender, followed by your 1 tablespoon of mayonnaise and your 1/2 teaspoon of salt.
5. Blend for about 1 minute before pouring the blended ingredients into your casserole dish.
6. Drizzle your 2 tablespoons of melted butter on top and stick the dish into the oven
7. Cook for 15 minutes. Serve when ready.

Nutrition:

Calories 67

Fat 3g

Carbohydrates 9g

Protein 2g

92. Vegan Lentil Burger

Preparation Time: 10 minutes

Cooking Time: 2 hours

Servings: 6

Ingredients:

- Brown lentils 3/4 cup
- Extra-virgin olive oil 2 teaspoons
- Low-sodium vegetable broth or water 1and3/4 cups
- Red onion, half thinly sliced, and half chopped 1 large
- Juice of half lemon
- Kosher salt
- Fresh spinach 8 ounces
- Garlic cloves, minced 2 larges
- Black pepper
- Ground cumin, half teaspoon
- Whole-wheat breadcrumbs 1 cup
- Cooking spray
- Walnuts, toasted and finely chopped half cup
- Whole-grain vegan buns 6

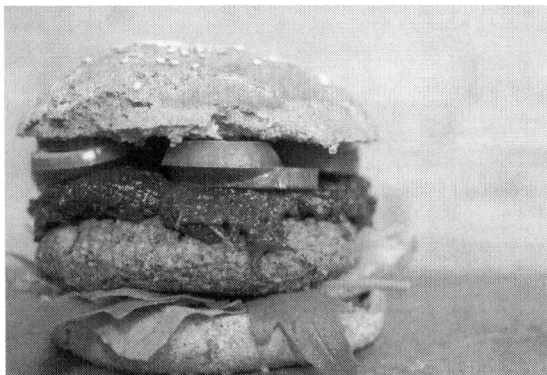

Directions:

1. Take the lentils and 1 3/4 cup of the broth for boiling at high temperature in a medium saucepan.
2. Decrease heat to medium-low, partly covered, and cook until the lentils are entirely softened. The liquid is absorbed for around 30 minutes.
3. Mix it with the leftover one tablespoon of the broth and mix well with the stick blender. Set it aside.
4. Warm the oil over medium temperature in a large nonstick skillet. Add the lemon juice, chopped onion, and 1/4 teaspoon salt and cook for around 6 minutes, stirring till soft.

5. Add the spinach, garlic, 1 and a half teaspoons of black pepper, and cumin and stir until the spinach is withered for around 3 minutes.
6. Add the mixture of spinach, breadcrumbs, walnuts, and salt to the lentils and blend thoroughly. Put a cover and refrigerate for at least one hour or overnight.
7. Heat the grill to medium-high. Shape the mixture into six 4-inch patties and sprinkle each side with a cooking spray.
8. Grill till pleasant grill marks are formed, around 3 minutes per hand.
9. Put the patties in the buns with the chopped onion and other seasonings and eat.

Nutrition:

Calories 177

Fat 3g

Carbohydrates 29g

Protein 9g

93.   Veggie-stuffed Omelet

Preparation Time: 10 minutes

Cooking Time: 30 minutes

Servings: 1

Ingredients:

- 2 eggs, beaten
- 1/4 cup mushrooms, sliced
- 1 cup loosely packed contemporary
- 1 baby spinach leaves, rinsed
- 2 tablespoons red bell pepper, chopped
- 1 tablespoon onion, chopped
- 1 tablespoon reduced-fat cheddar cheese, shredded
- 1 teaspoon olive or canola oil
- 1 tablespoon water
- 1/2 tsp. salt
- 1/2 tsp. pepper

Directions:

1. Warm the oil in a nonstick skillet. Sauté the mushrooms, onion, and bell pepper for about 2 minutes until the onion is tender.
2. Put the spinach and continue to cook, frequently stirring, until the spinach wilts. Once cooked, transfer the vegetables to a small bowl.
3. In a medium bowl, whisk the beaten eggs, water, salt, and pepper until well combined.
4. Place the same skillet in which you cooked the vegetable mixture over medium-high heat. Add the egg mixture immediately.
5. Make a quick, sliding back-and-forth motion with the pan, using a spatula to spread the eggs at the bottom of the pan.
6. Once the mixture is applied, let it stand for a few seconds to brown the bottom of the omelet lightly. Do not overcook it.
7. Carefully place the vegetable mixture on the half side of the omelet.
8. Top it with cheese and, using a spatula, gently fold the other half over the vegetables. Transfer the veggie-stuffed omelet to a plate and serve.

Nutrition:

Calories 150   Fat 8g   Carbohydrates 8g   Protein 24g

94.   Kamut Savory Salad

Preparation Time: 10 minutes
Cooking Time: 20 minutes
Servings: 5
Ingredients:
- 1 cup Kamut grain, soaked in water overnight, drained
- 1/4 cup frozen mixed vegetables
- 1 small carrot, chopped
- 1/2 cup mixed bell pepper, chopped
- 1 small onion, chopped
- 1/4 cup canned red kidney beans (alternative: cooked beans)
- 1 tsp olive oil
- 3 cups vegetable stock
- salt to taste
- pepper to taste
- Spring onion, to garnish
- parsley, to garnish

Directions:
1. Add Kamut and stock into a saucepan. Place a saucepan over medium heat. Cook until tender. Set aside.
2. Place a pan over medium heat. Add oil. When heated, put onion and sauté until translucent.
3. Add the rest of the ingredients and stir. Heat thoroughly.
4. Sprinkle spring onions and parsley to garnish.

Nutrition:
Calories 170
Fat 8g
Carbohydrates 8g
Protein 4g

95.   Freekeh Salad

Preparation Time: 10 minutes

Cooking Time: 10 minutes

Servings: 2

Ingredients:

- 2 vine tomatoes, chopped or 4 cherry tomatoes, quartered
- Sea salt to taste
- 2 tbsp olive oil
- Juice of 1/2 lemon
- Zest of 1/2 lemon, grated
- 1 fresh cilantro or parsley, chopped
- 1 small cucumber, chopped
- 1/2 cup corn kernels
- 1 small onion, chopped
- 3/4 cup freekeh
- 2 cups water

To serve:

- Hummus or pesto as required
- Avocado slices
- Mini tortillas or wraps, as required

Directions:

1. Add freekeh and water. Place water with medium heat.
2. Once boiling, lower the heat and cover with a lid.
3. Simmer for 10-12 minutes. Uncover and cook until tender. Drain and set aside.
4. Add lemon juice, oil, zest, salt, and pepper into a small bowl and whisk well.
5. Put the rest of the ingredients, including freekeh, into a bowl and toss well. Pour dressing on top and toss well. Chill until ready to use.
6. Spread tortillas on your countertop. Place salad on one-half of the tortillas. Top with avocado and hummus. Fold over the filling and serve.

Nutrition:

Calories 150   Fat 10g   Carbohydrates 22g   Protein 6g

96.   Poached Egg with Spinach

Preparation time: 5
minutes
Cooking time: 5
minutes
Servings: 1
Ingredients:

- 1 tablespoon.
  rice vinegar
- 2 egg
- 2 slices of soy
  bread
- 2 tbsp lumpfish roe
- 2 cups of spinach
- 1 tbsp extra virgin olive oil
- Salt
- Black pepper

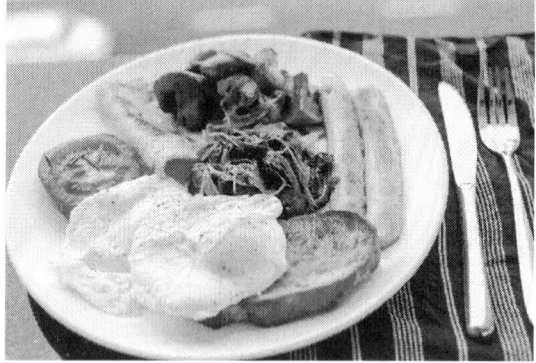

Directions:

1. Put some water in a saucepan and heat.
2. Simmer add vinegar and mix.
3. Break the egg into boiling water and cook for 4 minutes, making sure it stays in a compact form.
4. Warm oil in a saucepan and cook the spinach with the lid on 5 min.
5. Toast the bread.
6. Put the slices of bread on the plate and place the well-squeezed spinach on top.
7. Transfer the egg to the slices of bread and sprinkle with the lumpfish eggs.

Nutrition:
Calories 200
Fat 8g
Carbohydrates 8g
Protein 6g

97.   Tofu and Green Bean Stir-Fry

Preparation Time: 15 minutes

Cooking Time: 20 minutes

Servings: 4

Ingredients:

- 1 (14-ounce) package extra-firm tofu
- 2 tablespoons canola oil
- 1-pound green beans, chopped
- 2 carrots, peeled and thinly sliced
- 1/2 cup Stir-Fry Sauce or store-bought lower-sodium stir-fry sauce
- 2 cups Fluffy Brown Rice
- 2 scallions, thinly sliced
- 2 tablespoons sesame seeds

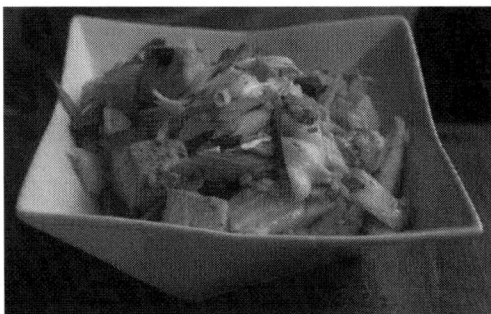

Directions:

1. Put the tofu on your plate lined with a kitchen towel.
2. Put another kitchen towel over the tofu, and place a heavy pot on top, changing towels every time they become soaked.
3. Let sit within 15 minutes to remove the moisture. Cut the tofu
4. Heat the canola oil in a large wok or skillet to medium-high heat.
5. Add the tofu cubes and cook, flipping every 1 to 2 minutes, so all sides become browned.
6. Remove from the skillet and place the green beans and carrots in the hot oil.
7. Stir-fry for 4 to 5 minutes, occasionally tossing, until crisp and slightly tender.
8. While the vegetables are cooking, prepare the Stir-Fry Sauce (if using homemade).
9. Place the tofu back in the skillet. Put the sauce over the tofu and vegetables and let simmer for 2 to 3 minutes.
10. Serve over rice, then top with scallions and sesame seeds.

Nutrition:

Calories: 218   Fat: 11g   Carbohydrates: 20g   Protein: 12g

98.   Peanut Vegetable Pad Thai

Preparation Time: 15 minutes

Cooking Time: 20 minutes

Servings: 6

Ingredients:

- 8 ounces brown rice noodles
- 1/3 cup natural peanut butter
- 3 tablespoons unsalted vegetable broth
- 1 tablespoon low-sodium soy sauce
- 2 tablespoons of rice wine vinegar
- 1 tablespoon honey
- 2 teaspoons sesame oil
- 1 teaspoon sriracha (optional)
- 1 tablespoon canola oil
- 1 red bell pepper, thinly sliced
- 1 zucchini, cut into matchsticks
- 2 large carrots, cut into matchsticks
- 3 large eggs, beaten
- 3/4 teaspoon kosher or sea salt
- 1/2 cup unsalted peanuts, chopped
- 1/2 cup cilantro leaves, chopped

Directions:

1. Boil a large pot of water. Cook the rice noodles as stated in package directions.
2. Mix the peanut butter, vegetable broth, soy sauce, rice wine vinegar, honey, sesame oil, and sriracha in a bowl. Set aside.
3. Warm-up canola oil over medium heat in a large nonstick skillet. Add the red bell pepper, zucchini, and carrots, and sauté for 2 to 3 minutes, until slightly soft.
4. Stir in the eggs and fold with a spatula until scrambled. Add the cooked rice noodles, sauce, and salt.
5. Toss to combine. Spoon into bowls and evenly top with the peanuts and cilantro.

Nutrition:

Calories: 393   Fat: 19g   Carbohydrates: 38g   Protein: 13g

99.   Sweet Potato Cakes with Classic Guacamole

Preparation Time: 15 minutes

Cooking Time: 20 minutes

Servings: 4

Ingredients:

For the guacamole:

- 2 ripe avocados, peeled and pitted
- 1/2 jalapeño, seeded and finely minced
- 1/4 red onion, peeled and finely diced
- 1/4 cup fresh cilantro leaves, chopped
- Zest and juice of 1 lime
- 1/4 teaspoon kosher or sea salt

For the cakes:

- 3 sweet potatoes, cooked and peeled
- 1/2 cup cooked black beans
- 1 large egg
- 1/2 cup panko breadcrumbs
- 1 teaspoon ground cumin
- 1 teaspoon chili powder
- 1/2 teaspoon kosher or sea salt
- 1/4 teaspoon ground black pepper
- 2 tablespoons canola oil

Directions:

1. Mash the avocado, then stir in the jalapeño, red onion, cilantro, lime zest and juice, and salt in a bowl. Taste and adjust the seasoning, if necessary.
2. Put the cooked sweet potatoes plus black beans in a bowl and mash until paste forms.
3. Stir in the egg, breadcrumbs, cumin, chili powder, salt, and black pepper until combined.
4. Warm-up canola oil in a large skillet at medium heat. Form the sweet potato mixture into 4 patties, place them in the hot skillet, and cook within 3 to 4 minutes per side until browned and crispy.
5. Serve the sweet potato cakes with guacamole on top.

Nutrition: Calories: 300   Fat: 15g   Carbohydrates: 42g   Protein: 4g

100. Lentil Avocado Tacos

Preparation Time: 15 minutes
Cooking Time: 35 minutes
Servings: 6
Ingredients:

- 1 tablespoon canola oil
- 1/2 yellow onion, peeled and diced
- 2-3 garlic cloves, minced
- 11/2 cups dried lentils
- 1/2 teaspoon kosher or sea salt
- 3 to 31/2 cups unsalted vegetable or chicken stock
- 21/2 tablespoons Taco Seasoning or store-bought low-sodium taco seasoning
- 16 (6-inch) corn tortillas, toasted
- 2 ripe avocados, peeled and sliced

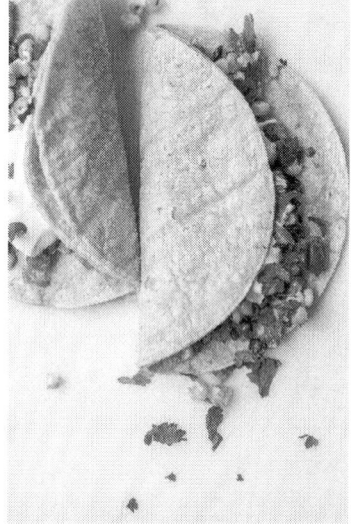

Directions:

1. Heat up the canola oil in a large skillet or Dutch oven over medium heat. Cook the onion within 4 to 5 minutes, until soft.
2. Mix in the garlic and cook within 30 seconds until fragrant. Then add the lentils, salt, and stock. Bring to a simmer for 25 to 35 minutes, adding additional stock if needed.
3. When there's only a small amount of liquid left in the pan, and the lentils are al dente, stir in the taco seasoning and let simmer for 1 to 2 minutes.
4. Taste and adjust the seasoning, if necessary. Spoon the lentil mixture into tortillas and serve with the avocado slices.

Nutrition:
Calories: 304
Fat: 10g
Carbohydrates: 44g
Protein: 9g

101. Black-Bean and Vegetable Burrito

Preparation Time: 15 minutes

Cooking Time: 15 minutes

Servings: 4

Ingredients:

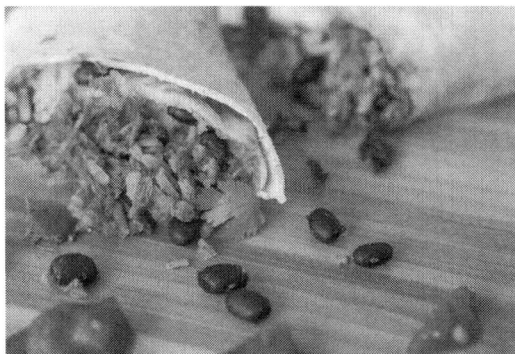

- 1/2 tablespoon olive oil
- 2 red or green bell peppers, chopped
- 1 zucchini or summer squash, diced
- 1/2 teaspoon chili powder
- 1 teaspoon cumin
- Freshly ground black pepper
- 2cans black beans drained and rinsed
- 1 cup cherry tomatoes, halved
- 4 (8-inch) whole-wheat tortillas
- Optional for serving spinach, sliced avocado, chopped scallions, or hot sauce

Directions:

1. Warm the oil in a large sauté pan over medium heat.
2. Add the bell peppers and sauté until crisp-tender, about 4 minutes.
3. Add the zucchini, chili powder, cumin, and black pepper to taste, and continue to sauté until the vegetables are tender about 5 minutes.
4. Add the black beans and cherry tomatoes and cook within 5 minutes.
5. Divide between 4 burritos and serve topped with optional ingredients as desired. Enjoy immediately.

Nutrition:

Calories: 290

Fat: 8g

Carbohydrates: 45g

Protein: 8g

102. Beet Blast Smoothie

Preparation Time: 5 minutes
Cooking Time: 5 minutes
Servings: 1
Ingredients:

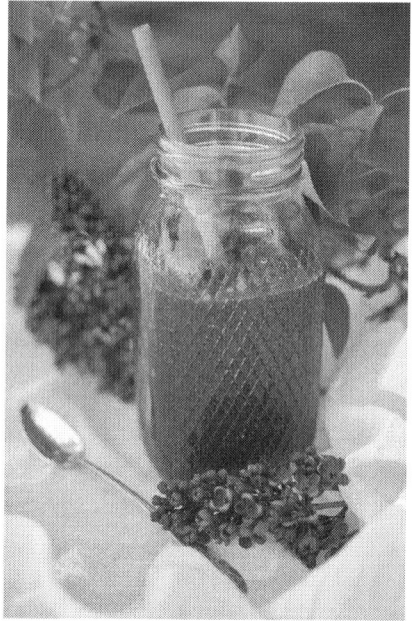

- 1 1/2 cups unsweetened plant-based milk
- 1 apple, peeled, cored, and chopped (preferably Granny Smith)
- 1 cup chopped frozen beets
- 1 cup frozen blueberries
- 1/2 cup frozen cherries
- 1/4-inch fresh ginger root, peeled

Directions:

1. Prepare all the ingredients in a blender and combine until smooth.
2. Serve immediately or store in the freezer in a resalable jar.

Nutrition:

Calories: 230
Fat: 2g
Carbohydrates: 54g
Protein: 5g

103. Green Power Smoothie

Preparation Time: 5 minutes
Cooking Time: 5 minutes
Servings: 1
Ingredients:
- 3 cups fresh spinach
- 11/2 cups frozen pineapple
- 1 cup unsweetened plant-based milk
- 1 cup fresh kale
- 1 apple, peeled, cored, and chopped
- 1/2 small avocado, pitted and peeled
- 1/2 teaspoon spirulina
- 1 tablespoon hemp seeds

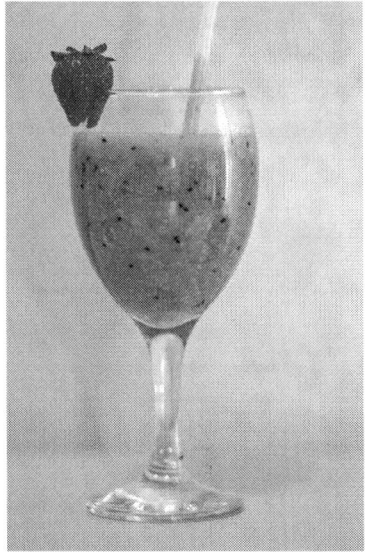

Directions:
1. Prepare all the ingredients in the blender and mix until smooth.
2. Serve immediately or store in the freezer in a resalable jar.

Nutrition:
Calories: 320
Fat: 0g
Carbohydrates: 65g
Protein: 27g

104. Tropical Bliss Smoothie

Preparation Time: 5 minutes
Cooking Time: 5 minutes
Servings: 1
Ingredients:

- 2 cups frozen pineapple
- 1 banana
- 1 1/4 cups unsweetened coconut milk
- 1/4 cup frozen coconut pieces
- 1/2 teaspoon ground flaxseed
- 1 teaspoon hemp seeds

Directions:

1. Prepare all the ingredients in the blender and mix until smooth.
2. Serve immediately or store in the freezer in a resalable jar.

Nutrition:

Calories: 351
Fat: 0g
Carbohydrates: 29g
Protein: 26g

105. Berry Antioxidant Smoothie

Preparation Time: 5 minutes
Cooking Time: 5 minutes
Servings: 1
Ingredients:

- 1 banana
- 1 1/4 cups unsweetened plant-based milk
- 1/2 cup frozen strawberries
- 1/2 cup frozen blueberries
- 1/2 cup frozen raspberries
- 3 pitted Medjool dates
- 1 tablespoon hulled hemp seeds
- 1/2 tablespoon ground flaxseed
- 1 teaspoon ground chia seeds

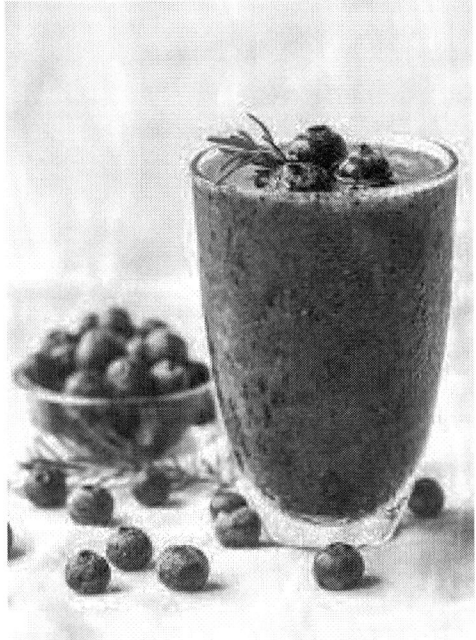

Directions:

1. Prepare all the ingredients in the blender and mix until smooth.
2. Serve immediately or store in the freezer in a resalable jar.

Nutrition:
Calories: 278
Fat: 15g
Carbohydrates: 36g
Protein: 2g

Chapter 9.   Frequently Asked Questions

It's important to have the correct information if you're contemplating or following intermittent fasting.

You'll be more able to fast correctly if you have the details. And if you fast correctly, you'll be more likely to see the weight loss, stable energy, and decreased cravings that have rendered intermittent fasting increasingly successful.

There are many fasting styles, all of which have been shown to improve physical wellbeing and weight loss. Unfortunately, these advantages are often overwhelmed by myths and stereotypes that discourage many people from ever trying Intermittent Fasting.

Unfortunately, there are several misunderstandings about it. You've already heard things such as fasting causes the metabolism to slow down, fasting causes the muscles to shrivel up, and you shouldn't drink water when fasting.

Fasting myths, on the other hand, are not based on fact. Instead, they're established on rumor, speculation, and misplaced faith in conventional thinking.

Here are few myths about intermittent fasting debunked to get you on your way. Therefore, you will make more informed choices regarding intermittent fasting to enhance your wellbeing.

Can I Drink Liquids During the Fast?

Several reports have emerged claiming that no-water fasts are beneficial to one's fitness. However, due to the impact of fasting, limiting water can contribute to serious dehydration. That's why, when supervising patients that are on therapeutic fasts, doctors pay particular attention to fluid consumption.

Electrolytes, including sodium and potassium, which are also energetically excreted out during fasting, are often monitored by doctors. So, during a fast, drink plenty of water and take sodium and potassium supplements along with it if the fast lasts more than 13 or 14 hours.

Isn't It Unhealthy to Skip Breakfast?

Breakfast is thought to provide you with the energy boost you require to start your day. The body will adjust by increasing adrenaline levels (growth hormone) and cortisol if you don't eat first thing in the morning. It will cause the liver to release glucose, providing you with the energy you need to start your day. As a result, eating breakfast isn't that essential.

Breakfast is most often associated with eating in the morning. It is more socially appropriate to recognize that it does not matter when one breaks their overnight fast until the term is broken down (breakfast).

Can I Work Out While Fasted?

Intermittent fasting, when paired with proper practice and exercise, will help you lose weight. Nevertheless, anyone following the diet should be aware that performing so independently is not a magical way to lose weight.

Don't take your health and welfare for granted; they are aspects that you would strive hard to sustain throughout your life. Fasting won't offer you the perfect body immediately, while if you do lose weight, you'll have to maintain it with healthier routines like eating well and exercising more.

Will Fasting Cause Muscle Loss?

It's been suggested that you'd have to fast for five days or more until any considerable amount of muscle is used for energy. Muscle tissue is constantly broken down and replaced and fasting will assist this mechanism by encouraging autophagy or the clearance of old proteins in favor of newer ones; less likely to be weakened – a positive thing. Fasting paired with resistance exercise has been shown to improve efficiency and muscle building of worked muscle. Fasting increases growth hormones, which may justify some of this.

Will Fasting Slow Down My Metabolism?

If you're scared that your metabolism will slow down by intermittent fasting, then it's a myth, and here is a logic to disprove it. Intermittent fasting isn't about limiting calories; it's about restricting time when to consume these calories.

There is no difference in metabolic rate if you wait a couple of hours longer to consume your first meal. Undereating causes physiological changes like metabolic rate, which do not arise while following an intermittent fasting diet.

Intermittent fasting is only one of the food approaches that will help you boost your health in various ways. It encourages both a stable and strong mind and body, and it's far more than just weight reduction. If one is worried that their new nutritional approach is not helping them meet their fitness objectives, none of the debunked misconceptions can deter them from pursuing Intermittent Fasting.

Conclusion

Thank you for reading this book. I hope it's helpful for you. Keep in mind that intermittent fasting for over 50 is not a quick-fix diet to lose weight but rather a lifestyle change. Do not stop if you do not lose weight after the first week. Keep going, be consistent with it, and eventually, you will achieve your goals.

It can sometimes be hard to get through the first week if it is your first time trying intermittent fasting. If you think you cannot do it, maybe it's because your body is not used to this yet. However, you can stick with the program and keep it ongoing. Before you know it, your body will get used to it, and adapting wouldn't be a problem anymore.

This guide includes healthy recipes for women over 50 that will surely keep your body energized and happy. These recipes are based on an intermittent fasting plan for women over 50.

It is very easy to follow, hassle-free, and you do not often visit the grocery. It is also cheaper. You do not have to buy food that is easy to prepare and cook at home because you can easily make it. You will have more time to do what you love to do, and that is, of course, spending time with your loved ones.

By implementing this guide into your daily life, you will control your blood sugar levels, control your cholesterol levels, and lose unwanted body fat.

Intermittent fasting for over 50 is a way to achieve overall health benefits. It can be easy to get into and maintain this type of lifestyle with a proper diet plan. It also promotes longevity in old age and a better quality of life.

It is recommended to eat healthy foods three to six times per day and make sure you get exercise at least three days a week. Additionally, make sure you drink at least eight glasses more water a day.

Try not to go too hungry in between meals, especially when you start your new lifestyle. Also, try to avoid eating the same kind of food all the time. It is important to have variety. Introduce new foods and cuisines to your diet. Make sure the foods you eat are healthy. This will help you maintain a good balance in your diet.

If you choose to incorporate intermittent fasting for over 50 into your lifestyle, remember that it is a lifestyle change, not a diet change. It will take time for your body to adjust, but most people find it easier than expected. So, take it slow and do not give up. The benefits you will get from this lifestyle change are endless.

Long-term weight loss is a hard thing to achieve. The rate of change and success varies from person to person. Take your time when it comes to dieting, and therefore there are so many diets. Intermittent fasting for over 50 is an effective way of losing weight quickly, but it is not easy. Set small goals to achieve and achieve them one step at a time.

Intermittent fasting for women over 50 does require some effort, but it can be an effective way to improve your diet and achieve better health in general. It is also very important that you remain consistent with it. It will motivate you to continue even more once you see results.

Made in the USA
Columbia, SC
20 October 2021